HANDBOOK OF

DIAGNOSTIC ENDOCRINOLOGY

To: Georgette Zoltani

Best Wishes!

Danny W. Chan
1999

HANDBOOK OF DIAGNOSTIC ENDOCRINOLOGY

EDITED BY

ISHWARLAL JIALAL, MD, PHD, FRCPATH, DABCC

WILLIAM E. WINTER, MD, DABCC

DANIEL W. CHAN, PHD, DABCC

AACC

AACC Press • 2101 L Street, NW, Suite 202 • Washington, DC 20037-1526

ISBN 1-890883-08-5

Printed in the United States of America

Dedication

This book is dedicated to our mentors, fellows, students and most of all to our wives, Jeanita, Nancy Hardt and Maria, and children, Rohan, Romini, Ganesh, Katie, Will, and Jackie, for their unselfish support, sacrifices, and continuing encouragement. The editors also express their gratitude to Joanna Grimes, John Gill, and AACC Press for their major effort in bringing this venture to fruition.

Ishwarlal Jialal
William E. Winter
Daniel W. Chan

Dedication

Contents

Contributors

Daniel D. Bankson, S.M., Ph.D., DABCC
Chief, Special Chemistry and STAT Laboratories
Veterans Affairs Puget Sound Health Care System
Assistant Clinical Professor
Department of Laboratory Medicine
University of Washington
Seattle, Washington

Daniel W. Chan, Ph.D., DABCC, FACB
Director, Clinical Chemistry Division
Associate Professor of Pathology, Oncology, Urology and Radiology
Johns Hopkins Medical Institutions
Baltimore, Maryland

Laurence M. Demers, Ph.D., DABCC
Distinguished Professor, Pathology and Medicine
The Pennsylvania State University College of Medicine
The PennState Geisinger Health System
Hershey, Pennsylvania

Gary W. Edelson, M.D., F.A.C.E.
Associate Professor of Medicine
Division of Endocrinology
Wayne State University School of Medicine
Detroit, Michigan

Carolyn S. Feldkamp, Ph.D.
Section Head, Immunochemistry
Chemistry Division
Department of Pathology
Henry Ford Hospital
Detroit, Michigan

Ishwarlal Jialal, M.D., Ph.D., FRCPath, DABCC
Director, Division of Clinical Biochemistry and Human Metabolism
Associate Director, Division of Clinical Pathology
Professor of Pathology and Internal Medicine
University of Texas, Southwestern Medical Center
Dallas, Texas

Rattan Juneja, M.B.B.S., M.D., MRCP
Resident, Department of Medicine
Veterans Affairs Puget Sound Health Care System
University of Washington
Seattle, Washington

Michael Kleerekoper, M.D., F.A.C.E.
Professor of Medicine
Division of Endocrinology
Wayne State University School of Medicine
Detroit, Michigan

Lori J. Sokoll, Ph.D.
Clinical Chemist
Department of Pathology
The Johns Hopkins Medical Institutions
Baltimore, Maryland

William E. Winter, M.D.
Professor
Departments of Pathology, Laboratory Medicine & Immunology, Pediatrics, and Molecular Genetics & Microbiology
Medical Director and Section Chief, Clinical Chemistry
Program Director, Pathology Residency Training Program
University of Florida College of Medicine
Gainesville, Florida

M. Saeed Zafar, M.D.
Endocrinology and Metabolism Division
Department of Internal Medicine
Henry Ford Hospital
Detroit, Michigan

Introduction

I. JIALAL, W. WINTER & D. CHAN

Both endocrine and metabolic disorders are significant causes of morbidity and mortality. Advances in protein chemistry, cellular and molecular biology, and genetics have resulted in a better appreciation of the etiology and pathophysiology of endocrine and metabolic disorders. Endocrine and metabolic disorders can be broadly classified as syndromes of excess, deficiency, and hormone resistance. It is abundantly clear that the most objective data for the diagnosis and management of these disorders derive from the clinical laboratory. From the initial days of radioimmunoassay, hormones can now readily be measured using non-isotopic technology (fluorescence, enzymes and luminescence). These assays are now available at most major medical centers and hospitals, largely in the form of heterogenous assays on automated analyzers, and thus provide a rapid turnaround time. This has clearly facilitated our approach to the diagnosis and management of endocrine and metabolic disorders.

There appears to be a lack of a readily available guide for clinical chemists, clinical pathologists, medical technologists, and endocrinologists to aid in the investigation and management of these disorders. The editors recognized a need to provide a readily available handbook that would mainly cover the laboratory aspects of endocrine and metabolic disorders. Thus, the purpose of this book is to bridge this gap and provide a handy reference for the diagnosis of endocrine and metabolic disorders. While it is not possible to cover all endocrine and metabolic disorders comprehensively, it is the task of the editors to confine this book to those endocrine disorders for which the laboratory plays a pivotal role in their diagnosis and management. Thus, in addition to covering the more common disorders such as hyperlipidemia, diabetes mellitus, thyroid disorders and metabolic bone disease, this book also reviews less common disorders of the endocrine system (such as disorders of the adrenal gland and pituitary gland, endocrine disorders of the gastrointestinal tract, and malignancy-associated endocrine disorders) and reproductive endocrinology.

In each chapter, the major focus is on the biochemical tests that are required either in the basal state or following provocation or suppression to help in the diagnosis of the relevant disorder. In addition to emphasizing the laboratory diagnosis, a review of the relevant physiology, biochemistry and the clinical syndrome is presented before the laboratory investigation is detailed. Also, as appropriate, in addition to plasma/serum assays for hormones, measurement of hormones/metabolites in urine is reported, e.g., metanephrines in pheochromocytoma, urine free cortisol in Cushing syndrome, etc. With regards to the specific biochemical test for the appropriate disorder, the value of the hormone assay in the basal state as well as following provocation or suppression is detailed. For example, in the diagnosis of adrenal insufficiency the cosyntropin test and its interpretation are described. For the diagnosis of prolactinoma, measurement of basal prolactin levels is emphasized. In the diagnosis of Cushing syndrome both basal tests, such as urine free cortisol, and the value of provocative tests, such as dexamethasone suppression tests, are presented. Also, where appropriate, the recent advances in molecular diagnostics have been incorporated, such as screening for the RET-proto-oncogene mutations for multiple endocrine neoplasia type II and medullary carcinoma of the thyroid and apoE genotyping for type III dyslipidemia, etc.

The editors have chosen to focus on the following disorders in this book: disorders of the pituitary gland, disorders of the thyroid gland, adrenal gland disorders, reproductive endocrinology, disorders of mineral metabolism, diabetes mellitus/hypoglycemia, hyperlipidemia, endocrine disorders of the gastrointestinal tract and malignancy-associated endocrine disorders. It is hoped that this book will provide a valuable addition to existing textbooks of endocrinology since it specifically fills the gap in the area of diagnostic endocrinology. Since endocrine and metabolic disorders constitute a major part of the workload of clinical laboratories, the major focus of this book was to provide a guide to laboratorians (clinical chemists, clinical pathologists, medical technologists, etc.) to help them better appreciate the various assays performed in the laboratory and their interpretation. Also, we believe that, given the changing trends in health care, directors of clinical laboratories will function increasingly as consultants to primary care physicians with regard to the investigation of certain disorders. This is particularly true with regard to endocrine and metabolic disorders.

I

Laboratory Investigation of Disorders of the Pituitary Gland

ISHWARLAL JIALAL, MD, PHD, FRCPATH, DABCC

A. Anterior Pituitary

Physiology and biochemistry

The hormones secreted by the anterior pituitary include the peptide hormones growth hormone (GH), prolactin (PRL) and adrenocorticotropin (ACTH) and the glycoprotein hormones thyroid-stimulating hormone (TSH) and the gonadotropins—luteinizing hormone (LH) and follicle-stimulating hormone (FSH). Hormonal synthesis and secretion by the anterior pituitary is controlled by the hypothalamus via hypophysiotropic hormones which, after reaching the anterior pituitary by the portal system, stimulate or inhibit the release of a given trophic hormone. Control of hypophysiotropic secretion is complex and comes in part from chemical and neuronal inputs from higher brain centers. The hypophysiotropic regulation of the anterior pituitary is shown in Table I. The hypothalamus serves as a relay station which receives chemical messages from higher

TABLE 1. HYPOTHALAMIC REGULATION OF THE ANTERIOR PITUITARY

HYPOTHALAMUS	EFFECT	PITUITARY CELL TYPE (HORMONE)	TARGET GLAND PRODUCT OR EFFECT
CRF	+	Corticotroph (ACTH)	Cortisol
GnRH *	+	Gonadotroph (LH and FSH)	Testosterone Estradiol
GHRH	+	Somatotroph (GH)	IGF-1
TRH	+	Thyrotroph (TSH)	Thyroxine & Triiodothyronine
SRIF (Somatostatin)	-	Somatotroph (GH)	IGF-1
Dopamine	-	Lactotroph (PRL)	Milk secretion

* *previously referred to as LHRH*

brain centers and feedback information from target glands upon which the pituitary hormones act. The hypothalamus then integrates these messages before it exerts its effect. These axes are described as closed-loop or negative feedback systems since hormones of target glands modulate hypothalamo-pituitary function.

Thyrotropin-releasing hormone (TRH) is a tripeptide which stimulates the release of TSH primarily. Although TRH also stimulates PRL secretion, this is probably not a physiological response.

Gonadotropin-releasing hormone (GnRH) is a decapeptide which stimulates the release of both LH and FSH. In adults, more LH than FSH is released, while prior to puberty more FSH than LH is released. GnRH is secreted episodically resulting in pulsatile secretion of gonadotropins.

Somatostatin (somatotropin-release inhibiting factor [SRIF]), which is a 14 amino acid peptide, blocks GH secretion and the TSH response to TRH at the pituitary level.

Growth hormone-releasing hormone (GHRH) is a 44 amino acid peptide which specifically releases GH only.

Corticotropin-releasing hormone (CRH) is a 41 amino acid peptide which stimulates the secretion of β-lipotropin and ACTH, both of which are derived from a precursor molecule, pro-opiomelanocortin. Unlike the acute response seen with other hypophysiotropic hormones, ACTH and cortisol levels remain elevated for several hours following CRH release.

Dopamine is, to date, the most important physiological inhibitor of PRL secretion. There is no agonist for PRL secretion. In the absence of dopamine, lactotrophs spontaneously secrete PRL.

Previously, classical histological staining techniques classified the cells of the pituitary as acidophils, basophils and chromophobes.

Immunocytochemical techniques using the antisera specific for individual hormones and electron microscopy allow the cells of the anterior pituitary to be classified according to their secretory products.

Somatotrophs and lactotrophs are acidophils which secrete GH and PRL respectively. Thyrotrophs, corticotrophs and gonadotrophs are basophils which secrete TSH, ACTH and gonadotropins respectively. The remaining chromophobe cells do not stain immunocytochemically.

The main function of GH (a 191 amino acid polypeptide) is to stimulate linear growth. This effect is mediated by the somatomedins or insulin-like growth factors (IGFs), a group of small peptides produced by the liver and local tissues in response to GH, which stimulate protein synthesis. GH also directly stimulates lipolysis and has an antagonistic effect on insulin action. Its secretion is stimulated by sleep, exercise, stress (hypoglycemia), dopamine, certain amino acids, GHRH, ß-blockers, and glucagon. It is important to remember that GH is secreted in an episodic and pulsatile manner.

ACTH is a 39 amino acid peptide of which the first 24 amino acids are necessary for biological activity. While ACTH mainly stimulates the synthesis and secretion of glucocorticoids, it also has a minor effect on mineralocorticoids and adrenal androgens. ACTH is secreted in a pulsatile manner with a diurnal rhythm (highest secretion in early morning hours). While many types of stress, including hypoglycemia, stimulate ACTH release, ACTH secretion is inhibited by cortisol. Due to its melanocyte-stimulating action, excessive ACTH secretion can result in increased pigmentation.

TSH is a glycoprotein hormone with a molecular mass of 28,000 which stimulates the synthesis and secretion of thyroid hormones. Like LH and FSH, TSH is composed of two subunits: an α subunit and a β subunit. While TSH , LH, FSH and hCG all share the same α subunit, they have unique β subunits. TSH secretion is finely regulated by the levels of thyroid hormones in the blood and TRH.

PRL is a 198 amino acid polypeptide which is secreted under tonic inhibition by dopamine. The primary effect of PRL is the initiation and maintenance of lactation in the postpartum period. PRL is secreted in a pulsatile, episodic manner and its secretion is increased by stress, and in women it is dependent upon estrogen.

The gonadotropins (LH and FSH), like TSH, are glycoprotein hormones whose ß-subunit confers the biological and immunodiagnostic specificity of the hormone. Both LH and FSH have a molecular mass of 29000. In men, LH acts on Leydig cells to increase the synthesis and secretion of testosterone, while FSH (in concert with testosterone) acts on Sertoli cells to stimulate spermatogenesis. In women, LH stimulates estradiol and progesterone production by the ovary. A surge of LH in the mid-menstrual cycle is responsible for ovulation and continued LH secretion subsequently maintains the corpus luteum and progesterone production. Development of the ovarian follicle is largely under FSH control and the secretion of estradiol from this follicle is dependent on both LH and FSH. Both FSH and LH are under dual control of the hypothalamus and gonads. It has been shown that Sertoli cells and the ovary produce the hormone inhibin which suppresses FSH secretion. The gonadotropins are also secreted in an episodic manner. GnRH maintains basal gonadotropin secretion, generates the phasic release of gonadotropins for ovulation and determines the onset of puberty.

1. Hypopituitarism

Hypopituitarism is defined as a deficiency of either one or many pituitary hormones. Isolated hormone deficiency (monohypopituitarism) is usually due to a hypothalamic disorder while multiple hormone deficiency (panhypopituitarism) can result from disorders of both the pituitary and hypothalamus. Clinical manifestations of hypopituitarism are not evident until at least 75% of the pituitary gland is destroyed. Causes of hypopituitarism are shown in Table 2. The most common cause appears to be a pituitary tumor. In the postpartum period, hemorrhage leads to infarction of the vascular and enlarged pituitary gland resulting in hypopituitarism. This is referred to as Sheehan's syndrome. Sheehan's syndrome is an important cause of hypopituitarism, especially in developing countries.

In adults, **GH deficiency** has no obvious clinical manifestations but may contribute to the tendency to fasting hypoglycemia. However, the effect of GH replacement is under intense study presently. It is hoped that these studies will provide a solid rationale for GH replacement therapy. In children, longitudinal growth is severely retarded and height and growth rate fall below the 3rd percentile.

Secondary hypothyroidism resulting from **TSH deficiency** produces a similar picture to that of primary hypothyroidism with weakness, bradycardia, and delayed reflexes, except that the waxy infiltration of the subcutaneous tissue is less obvious.

TABLE 2. CAUSES OF HYPOPITUITARISM

Tumors - pituitary adenomas, craniopharyngiomas, metastatic carcinomas meningiomas, gliomas, and chordomas

Vascular disease - Sheehan's syndrome, vascular malformations, sickle cell disease, diabetes mellitus and pituitary apoplexy

Granulomas and infiltrative disorders - sarcoidosis, tuberculosis, syphilis, hemochromatosis, histiocytosis-X, lymphocytic hypophysitis

Trauma

Iatrogenic - surgery, irradiation, hormonal therapy

Miscellaneous - congenital absence of the pituitary, isolated hormone deficiencies

ACTH deficiency leads to adenocortical insufficiency characterized by decreased secretion of cortisol and adrenal androgens. The major clinical feature of ACTH deficiency is a tendency to spontaneous hypoglycemia. Unlike patients with primary hypoadrenalism who have hyperpigmentation, patients with ACTH deficiency have a pale skin. Furthermore, the renin-angiotensin-aldosterone axis is left essentially intact in patients who are ACTH deficient.

The major consequence of **PRL deficiency** is failure of lactation. This is usually seen in Sheehan's syndrome (postpartum pituitary necrosis) in which PRL deficiency is invariably accompanied by the other hormone deficiencies.

Deficiency of gonadotropins in children results in delayed or partial puberty. If GH secretion is intact, the patients have an eunuchoid habitus {tall with arm span> height and with the lower segment (pubis to ground) > upper segment (pubis to crown)} as the epiphyses have not fused. Isolated GnRH deficiency is more common in males and can be associated with midline defects, nerve deafness, color-blindness, and anosmia (Kallmann's syndrome). When GnRH deficiency occurs after puberty, clinical features in males include loss of libido, impotence, loss of secondary sex characteristics (facial, pubic, and axillary hair loss), and infertility (oligo- or azoospermia). Women may present with loss of libido, dyspareunia, loss of secondary sex characteristics, oligo-amenorrhoea and infertility.

Investigation of hypopituitarism

Depending upon the clinical setting, investigations should be directed to elucidate the cause. Routine investigation of patients suspected of having a tumor includes assessment of the visual fields and imaging studies of the pituitary fossa including computed tomography or magnetic resonance imaging (MRI). The preferred procedure is MRI. Initial biochemical screening to assess pituitary function includes measurement of TSH and free T4, PRL, LH, FSH, testosterone in males, and cortisol. The most useful test to diagnose TSH deficiency is serum free T4 since TSH levels can be low, normal, or high but biologically inactive. The diagnosis of secondary hypothyroidism can be difficult in the face of major illness since the sick euthyroid syndrome can have similar biochemical features. Ideally, a pooled sample (3 samples, 20 minutes apart) should be obtained for LH, FSH, prolactin, and testosterone. The best assessment of gonadotropin deficiency in premenopausal women is the menstrual history. Patients with hypothalamo-pituitary disease have low levels of both gonadotropins and sex hormones. A single estradiol level may be normal in women with hypogonadism. A useful index of ovulation is measurement of serum progesterone in the luteal phase since a value ≥5 ng/ml is supportive of ovulation. Men with gonadotropin deficiency have decreased levels of testosterone (total and free) with low or normal levels of FSH and LH. A semen analysis can also be undertaken.

A basal morning cortisol <5 μg/dL on two occasions confirms a diagnosis of hypoadrenalism. The most useful laboratory test to confirm a diagnosis of adrenal insufficiency is the rapid ACTH stimulation test. In this test cosyntropin (ACTH 1-24) is injected intramuscularly or intravenously at a dose of 250 μg and cortisol levels are obtained at baseline and 30 to 60 minutes following the injection. In normal subjects the basal cortisol is >6 μg/dL, the increment over basal is >7 μg/dL and the peak value is > 20μg/dL. A subnormal response is consistent with adrenocortical insufficiency. A plasma ACTH level and/or the clinical presentation of the patient will help delineate if it is primary or secondary. However, a normal response to cosyntropin does not rule out an impaired ACTH reserve (partial adrenal insufficiency) due to hypothalamo-pituitary disease. In order to rule out secondary hypoadrenalism certain other tests are required, such as the metyrapone test and insulin-induced hypoglycemia. Recent studies suggest that a low dose ACTH test (1 μg) provides similar information as the metyrapone and insulin-hypoglycemia tests in diagnosing ACTH deficiency. However, while this test shows promise and appears more sensitive in diagnosing ACTH deficiency, further studies are needed, especially in hospitalized patients, to establish its role. The simplest metyrapone test entails giving metyrapone (30 mg/kg) overnight and measuring plasma cortisol and 11-deoxycortisol the next morning. Metyrapone is given orally between 11-12 PM (2 g if weight <70 kg, 2.5 g if weight 79-90 kg, and 3 g if weight >90 kg) and plasma cortisol and 11-deoxycortisol are obtained at 8 AM the following morning. Metyrapone works by inhibiting 11β–hydroxylase and thus stimulating ACTH and 11-deoxycortisol secretion. Following metyrapone in normal subjects, the cortisol the next morning should be below 5 μg/dL and the 11-deoxycortisol levels should exceed 7 μg/dL.

Sometimes one needs to undertake the long metyrapone test. Metyrapone is given at a dose of 750 mg every 4 hours for 24 hours with 24-hour urine collections for 17 hydroxy corticosteriods (17-OHCS) before, during and for 24 hours after metyrapone. In normal individuals urinary 17-OHCS double, and if plasma 11 deoxycortisol is also measured, values in normals exceed 10 μg /dL. However, the overnight test is preferred because of its simplicity and lack of requirement for urine collection for steroids. A normal response to metyrapone denotes adequate function of the pituitary adrenal axis. A prolonged ACTH stimulation test (250 μg IV infusion over 8 hours per day for 3 days) can be useful since in patients with secondary hypoadrenalism there is a progressive rise in plasma cortisol to at least 20 μg/dL. However, the advent of reliable ACTH assays coupled with the rapid cosyntropin test and the overnight metyrapone test, are usually sufficient to diagnose ACTH deficiency. Insulin induced hypoglycemia can also be a useful test to rule out hypothalamo-pituitary disorders resulting in adrenal insufficiency.

The most popular approach to determine pituitary reserve was the triple bolus test. Briefly, in this test, TRH (500 μg), GnRH (100 μg), and insulin (0.05-0.15 U/kg body weight, dependent on insulin sensitivity) are injected intravenously and samples are obtained for LH, FSH, TSH, PRL, cortisol and GH. Samples for LH, FSH and TSH should be obtained at 0, 30 and 60 minutes. While this test assesses pituitary reserve comprehensively it is not commonly undertaken today. However, the cortisol and GH reserve can be adequately assessed by insulin-induced hypoglycemia over a 2-hour period by obtaining samples at 30 minute intervals. Following adequate hypoglycemia (≤40 mg/dL) or a 50% decrement from baseline, the cortisol and GH levels should exceed 20 μg/dL and 10 ng/mL respectively. In children with suspected GH deficiency, a screening test with either L-dopa, glucagon or exercise must be undertaken initially.

"Priming" patients for GH testing implies the administration of an agent prior to testing that will decrease the likelihood of a falsely abnormal (deficient) GH response. Priming should be performed before screening (e.g., exercise-stimulated GH testing) as well as definitive GH testing procedures. All preadolescent males (≥10 years old) should be primed. Although not absolutely necessary, it is also wise to prime girls undergoing GH testing. While one can use estrogen priming in boys and androgen priming in girls, it is most reasonable to use androgens in boys and estrogens in girls. Androgens are most commonly administered as testosterone enanthate 50 mg IM 2 to 3 weeks before the GH test. Large boys may require 100-200 mg of IM testosterone. Ethinyl estradiol, premarin, and diethylstilbesterol (DES) have been used as estrogen preparations. Patients <50 lb. receive 20 mg of ethinyl estradiol per dose 18, 12, and 1 hour prior to GH testing. Patients >50 lb. receive 50 mg per dose on the same schedule. Alternatively, 100 mg/day of ethinyl estradiol for 3 days prior to testing can be used. In patients <30 lb., 2.5 mg of premarin is used twice daily for 3 days. In patients ≥30 lb., 5 mg of premarin is used twice daily for 3 days. For DES, 5 mg per day for 3 days is employed prior to GH testing. Alternative protocols for priming that do not involve sex steroids include the use of propranolol in a dose of 0.5-0.75 mg/kg (maximum 40 mg), or, for children <20 kg, 20 mg 2 hrs pretest and, for children >20 kg, 40 mg 2 hrs pretest.

The GH response to certain secretagogues following an overnight fast can be used as screening tests to assess GH deficiency. The simplest test is to have the child exercise for 20 minutes and obtain a GH level 20 minutes later. GH also responds to the infusion of the amino acid L-arginine (0.5 g/kg IV over 30 minutes with a maximum dose of 30 g) with GH levels obtained at 30 minute intervals for 2 hours. This test is contraindicated with severe liver or renal disease and acidosis. During the L-dopa test GH levels are obtained at 30 minute intervals for 150 minutes following oral ingestion of L-dopa (125 mgs for up to 15 kg body weight, 250 mg for 15-30 kg and 500 mgs for >30 kg). The GH response to oral clonidine can also be used (0.1-0.15 mg/m2) orally. However, it can cause postural hypotension. A GH response ≥5 ng/ml during any of these tests makes GH deficiency a very unlikely diagnosis. Levels of both IGF-1 and its binding protein, IGF-BP-3, are dependent on GH secretion and are low with GH deficiency but may overlap into the reference range. Low levels of serum IGF-1 are confirmatory evidence of GH deficiency provided the patient is not malnourished, hypothyroid, chronically ill or elderly since all of these decrease IGF-1 levels.

The role of the GHRH test is to assess GH deficiency is evolving with wider availability of GHRH. Only if the GH response is inadequate (<5 ng/mL) with any of the above tests should one proceed to the insulin-induced hypoglycemia test. When hypoglycemia is contraindicated, e.g., with cortisol <5 µg/dL, seizure disorders and cerebrovascular or coronary artery disease, the glucagon test (1 mg intramuscularly) can be undertaken to assess GH and cortisol secretion at 30 minute intervals between 90 and 240 minutes. Based upon cost consideration, the added costs of TRH and GnRH tests cannot be justified in the routine workup of hypopituitarism. Anorexia nervosa, a psychological disorder characterized by self-imposed starvation and a preoccupation with body size, can resemble hypopituitarism since these patients have weight loss, amenorrhea and decreased gonadotropins. However, both cortisol and GH levels are increased.

2. Pituitary tumors

Pituitary tumors constitute the most common cause of hypopituitarism and they can be broadly classified into secretory and non-secretory tumors. They constitute about 10% of all intracranial neoplasms. In children, the most common tumor in the pituitary area is craniopharyngioma. Pituitary tumors may manifest themselves in many ways including local space-occupying effects (with bitemporal hemianopsia), hypopituitarism, hypersecretion of hormones or as an incidental radiological finding. Investigations (other than assessment of pituitary reserve) in patients with pituitary tumors include charting of visual fields and imaging studies of the pituitary fossa, such as computed tomography or magnetic resonance imaging. Tumors with a diameter of less than 10 mm are referred to as microadenomas.

Acromegaly

Increased secretion of GH prior to epiphyseal closure results in gigantism while in adults it results in acromegaly; both are usually due to a GH-producing pituitary adenoma. Gigantism is exceptionally rare. Other causes of acromegaly include ectopic GH or GHRH secretion in patients with carcinoids, islet cell tumors or lung carcinomas or eutopic GHRH secretion from a hypothalamic hamartoma. About 15% of tumors also contain lactotrophs and these tumors secrete both GH and PRL. Acral enlargement (skin, subcutaneous tissue and skeletal overgrowth), which is seen in all patients, is recognized by increasing ring, glove or shoe size. Other features include hyperhidrosis, hypertension, diabetes, cardiomyopathy, osteoarthritis, etc.

It should be remembered that rarely acromegaly may form part of the multiple endocrine neoplasia syndrome type I. The diagnosis of acromegaly is usually clinically obvious and can readily be confirmed by an assessment of GH secretion. Fasting plasma GH levels are > 5 ng/ml; however, single measurements are not reliable because of the pulsatile nature of GH secretion and other conditions such as anxiety, acute illness, anorexia nervosa, diabetes mellitus, cirrhosis, chronic renal failure, etc. can result in increased GH levels. The simplest and most specific test for confirming the diagnosis is the GH response to a 75 or 100 g oral glucose load. In normal subjects, GH levels are suppressed to <2 ng/mL (or <1 ng/mL with newer GH assays with good low end sensitivity) at 60 minutes while in acromegaly values do not suppress adequately; in fact, some patients may display a paradoxical rise. Another useful assay is measurement of IGF-1 level (somatomedin C) which is elevated in virtually all patients. In normal fed persons with normal renal and hepatic function, serum IGF-1 levels reflect the integrated effect of GH at the tissue level and correlates with 24-hr GH levels. Thus, IGF-1 levels provide an excellent screening test for acromegaly. It needs to be emphasized that IGF-1 reference ranges must be adjusted for age and sex. Other abnormalities observed in acromegaly include abnormal glucose tolerance, hyperprolactinaemia, hyperphosphataemia, hyperlipidemia, and hypercalcinuria. Criteria that constitute an adequate response to therapy include a fasting GH below 5 ng/mL, an adequate suppression following oral glucose (GH< 2ng/mL) and a normal IGF-1 level.

Prolactinomas

Prolactinomas are the most common secretory tumors of the pituitary and occur 8 times more frequently in women than in men. Tumor size varies greatly from microadenomas to large invasive macroadenomas with extrasellar extension. Female patients can present with galactorrhoea, amenorrhoea (usually secondary), loss of libido, anovulation, infertility and the local effects of tumor expansion. Males with prolactinomas may present with impotence, loss of libido, galactorrhoea, gynecomastia, infertility and the effects of tumor expansion. Hyperprolactinemia interferes with the normal pulsatile secretin of LH and FSH. Rarely, serum prolactin may be elevated because of macroprolactinemia. In this disorder, the increase in serum prolactin is due to a large molecular mass form that is immunoreactive but has reduced biologic activity. These patients have normal menses and fertility.

In patients with microadenomas, other pituitary functions are usually normal and basal testing of pituitary hormones will suffice. However, patients with macroadenomas should be assessed for hypopituitarism as already described. The most reliable tests for the diagnosis of a prolactinoma are several random measurements of PRL levels (preferably with pooled samples). It should be pointed out that prolactinomas are only one cause of hyperprolactinaemia. Table 3 shows the numerous causes; most of these (such as pregnancy, drugs, hypothyroidism or chronic renal failure) can be excluded by history, clinical examination and routine laboratory tests. Also, PRL levels are generally <100 ng/mL whereas PRL levels >100 ng/mL are usually caused by a prolactinoma, and levels >200 ng/mL are virtually diagnostic of prolactinoma. Provocative tests such as the TRH test have not proven useful in the diagnosis of prolactinomas.

TABLE 3. CAUSES OF HYPERPROLACTINAEMIA

Physiological - sleep, stress, pregnancy, lactation, newborn, nipple stimulation, exercise

Drugs - psychotropic agents such as phenothiazines, tricyclic antidepressants and opiate alkaloids; anti-emetics and antihistamines, e.g., metoclopramide, sulpiride, cimetidine; antihypertensives, e.g., methyldopa and reserpine; calcium channel blockers, hormones, e.g., oestrogens and TRH; monoamine oxidase inhibitors; butyrophenones

Hypothalamo-pituitary stalk lesions - craniopharyngioma, granulomas, stalk section following surgery, head injury or irradiation

Pituitary tumors - prolactinomas, mixed GH or ACTH and PRL adenomas

Miscellaneous - primary hypothyroidism, chronic renal failure, polycystic ovarian disease, idiopathic hyperprolactinaemia, liver disease, spinal cord lesions, macroprolactinemia, seizures

Other secretory tumors

The third most common secretory disorder of the pituitary is Cushing disease due to excess ACTH secretion; this is discussed in the chapter on adrenal disorders.

Pituitary tumors secreting glycoprotein hormones (TSH, LH, and FSH) are very uncommon. Clinically, TSH-secreting tumors present with hyperthyroidism, increased thyroxine levels with inappropriately elevated

TSH levels and increased α subunit levels with no TSH response to TRH. Gonadotropin-secreting tumors occur in males, the majority secreting FSH only, but tumors secreting both LH and FSH have been described. They are usually large chromophobe adenomas which present clinically with visual impairment, impotence and infertility. Patients have increased serum FSH and/or LH levels, and increased α subunit levels; testosterone levels are usually decreased or rarely increased due to increased secretion of bioactive LH.

Craniopharyngioma

Craniopharyngiomas develop from Rathke's pouch. They are suprasellar in location, non-secretory and the majority are cystic in nature. They are the most common pituitary tumors in children and young adults and can present with raised intracranial pressure, visual field defects and hypopituitarism (short stature, delayed puberty, diabetes insipidus, and hyperprolactinemia). Suprasellar calcification, which is present in over 70%, is a hallmark of this tumor. Suprasellar dysgerminomas can have a similar presentation and measurement of hCG in CSF can aid the diagnosis.

B. Posterior Pituitary

Both antidiuretic hormone (ADH) and oxytocin are synthesized in the cell bodies of the neurons of the supraoptic and paraventricular nuclei of the hypothalamus. After synthesis, ADH and its respective carrier protein, neurophysin, are packaged into neuro-secretory granules and then migrate along the axons of the neurons to the secretory terminals, where the hormones are stored. While most secretory terminals are in the posterior pituitary, others are at higher levels in the pituitary stalk and median eminence. The major action of ADH is to allow the urine to become concentrated in the collecting tubules by facilitating passive movement of water along the osmotic gradient from the lumen to the medullary interstitium. ADH release is mediated by osmotic and non-osmotic stimuli. The major determinant of ADH release is the plasma osmolality and this is mediated via osmoreceptors in the hypothalamus. A decrease in plasma volume also evokes ADH release. Other stimuli of ADH release include stress, nicotine, chlorpropamide, morphine, vincristine and barbiturates. To date, no clinical syndromes have been reported in patients with the absence of oxytocin. The two major disorders of ADH secretion are diabetes insipidus and the syndrome of inappropriate ADH secretion (SIADH).

Diabetes insipidus

Diabetes insipidus can result from either failure of ADH secretion (cranial or central) or failure of the kidneys to respond to ADH (nephrogenic). Permanent central diabetes insipidus will not develop until 80% of the pathways have been destroyed. Central diabetes insipidus is a rare disorder.

Causes of cranial diabetes insipidus are shown in Table 4. The most common form of diabetes insipidus is the idiopathic type, accounting for 30% of cases. Up to 40% of patients with the idiopathic variety have antibodies to ADH-secreting hypothalamic neurons. Rarely, diabetes insipidus (DI) is part of Wolfram's syndrome (DIDMOAD) which also includes diabetes mellitus (DM), optic atrophy (OA), and deafness (D). The presence of hypopituitarism and/or hyperprolactinema should prompt a search for a causative lesion by serial monitoring with imaging studies and hormone assays. During pregnancy, diabetes insipidus could result from increased placental degradation of ADH. This is termed gestational diabetes insipidus.

Table 4. Causes of Central Diabetes Insipidus

- Idiopathic
- Familial - dominant or recessive
- Trauma - head injury or surgery
- Tumors - pituitary tumors, craniopharyngioma or metastases
- Granulomas - sarcoidosis, histiocytosis, tuberculosis
- Infections - meningitis, encephalitis
- Vascular - Sheehan's syndrome, aneurysms, sickle cell anemia

The essential feature of diabetes insipidus is the elaboration of a large volume of dilute urine. The polyuria is of varying severity (3-15 L/day) and leads to hypertonic dehydration (hypernatremia with serum osmolality >295 mOsm/kg) which in turn stimulates the thirst mechanism, resulting in polydipsia with a craving for ice-water. Diabetes insipidus can sometimes be differentiated from psychogenic polydipsia since serum osmolality in the latter is low normal (≤280 mOsm/kg). If the patient with diabetes insipidus has free access to water, hypernatremia should not develop. However, if access to water is restricted or the patient has a damaged thirst center and doesn't drink, hypernatremia will develop.

A random urine osmolality which exceeds 750 mOsm/kg excludes diabetes insipidus. The most commonly used provocative test to diagnose this disorder is the water deprivation test. The water deprivation test should not be performed in the presence of hypothyroidism, adrenal insufficiency or if an osmotic diuresis is present, such as uncontrolled diabetes mellitus. Patients are deprived of all fluids until hourly urine osmolalities are constant (<30 mOsm/kg difference between consecutive samples) for 3 successive hours. At this point, a value for plasma osmolality is obtained and ADH administered. Desmopressin 1-2 mg subcutaneously or 10-20 µg intra-nasally is administered and urine osmolality is obtained at 60 minutes. In normal persons and patients with psychogenic polydipsia, urine osmolality is higher than plasma osmolality at the end of the dehydration and does not increase by more than 5% following ADH. Patients with partial diabetes insipidus have a urine osmolality greater than plasma osmolality (300 mOsm) following dehydration but urine osmolality increases by at least 9% following ADH. In severe diabetes insipidus, urine osmolality is less than plasma osmolality at the end of dehydration and increases by over 50% following ADH. The test should be terminated if body weight falls by more than 3%. If reliable ADH assays are available, plasma osmolality and ADH levels should be obtained following dehydration since relating these two variables will clearly differentiate cranial diabetes insipidus from other forms, as reported by Robertson, especially when osmolality measurements are inconclusive. In central DI, plasma ADH is subnormal relative to plasma osmolality following dehydration, while in nephrogenic DI plasma ADH is in the upper end of the reference range or elevated.

SIADH

SIADH is a disorder in which there is increased ADH secretion in spite of subnormal plasma osmolality. Water retention results in hyponatremia and serum hypo-osmolality but no edema. Suppression of aldosterone secretion and inhibition of proximal tubular sodium reabsorption and volume expansion lead to increased urinary sodium excretion. The main causes of SIADH are shown in Table 5. Most patients with SIADH do not have specific clinical features unless the hyponatremia is severe (Na^+ <125 mmol/L), when cerebral symptoms occur. Initial symptoms include anorexia, nausea, vomiting and headaches. With more severe hyponatremia ($Na^+ < 110$) or more rapidly developing hyponatremia, the symptoms of cerebral edema become evident such as irritability, confusion, disorientation, convulsions, hemiparesis, and coma.

TABLE 5. MAJOR CAUSES OF SIADH

Neoplasia - carcinoma of bronchus, duodenum, pancreas, bladder, ureter or prostate; lymphoma, thymoma, mesothelioma, Ewing's sarcoma

Pulmonary disorders - pneumonia, tuberculosis, lung abscess, positive pressure ventilation, chronic obstructive airway disease

CNS disorders - encephalitis, meningitis, head injury, Guillain-Barre syndrome, acute intermittent porphyria, brain abscess, brain tumor, subdural hematoma, subarachnoid hemorrhage, vasculitis (lupus)

Drugs - clofibrate, chlorpropamide, vincristine, cyclophosphamide, phenothiazines, tricyclic antidepressants, thiazides, carbamazepine, narcotics

The biochemical features which favor the diagnosis of SIADH include hyponatremia (Na^+ <120 mmol/L), low serum osmolality (< 280 mOsm/kg), low urea and uric acid, urine Na^+ >20 mmol/L, and urine osmolality (≥300 mOsm/kg) which exceeds plasma osmolality. Stricter criteria include the absence of dehydration, edema, adrenal insufficiency, hypothyroidism or renal failure.

In conclusion, there is a comprehensive array of tests that can be used to assess pituitary function. In some instances, basal hormone levels are adequate for diagnosis. In other instances provocative testing is needed. The biochemical evaluation of pituitary function detailed in this chapter is summarized in Table 6.

Table 6. Summary of Pituitary Hormone Assessment

HORMONE	DEFICIENCY	EXCESS
GH	GH response to arginine, exercise, L-Dopa or insulin. IGF-1 levels	IGF-1 levels, GH response to oral glucose (GTT)
PRL	PRL response TRH	basal PRL
TSH	T_4, TSH	T_4, TSH, alpha-subunit, TSH response to TRH
Gonadotropins	testosterone, estradiol, LH & FSH	LH, FSH, testosterone, alpha-subunit
ACTH	cortisol, cosyntropin test, metyrapone test, insulin tolerance test.	urine-free cortisol, overnight or low dose dexamethasone suppression tests
ADH	Water deprivation test (S&U osmol). ADH levels at maximum dehydration	S & U osmol S & U Na^+

S denotes Serum
U denotes Urine

References

1. Jialal I, Omar MAK, Nathoo BC, Mahabeer S. Disorders of the hypothalamus and pituitary gland. SA J Cont Med Educ 1987;5:25-33.
2. Vance ML. Hypopituitarism. N Engl J Med 1994;330(23):1651-1661.
3. Levy A, Lightman SL. Diagnosis and management of pituitary tumors. BMJ 1994;308:1087-1091.
4. Tyrrell JB, Aron DC, Findling JW. Hypothalamus & Pituitary. In: Basic and Clinical Endocrinology. FS Greenspan, JD Baxter, Appleton & Lange, Norwalk CT, 4th edition. 1994;64-127.
5. Jialal I, Norman R, Naidoo C. Pituitary function in Sheehan's syndrome. Obstet Gynecol 1984;63:15-19.
6. Robertson GL. Posterior Pituitary in Endocrinology and Metabolism by P. Felig, JD Baxter, and LA Frohman. 3rd edition. McGraw-Hill 1995 p 385-432.

7. Reichlin S, Thorner MO, Vance ML, Horvath E, Kovacs K, Reeves WB, Andreoli TE. Hypothalamus and Pituitary in Williams Textbook of Endocrinology, ed. JD Wilson and DW Foster, WB Saunders Co., Philadelphia 8th ed., 1992:135-356.
8. Frohman LA. Diseases of Anterior Pituitary in Endocrinology and Metabolism by P. Felig, JD Baxter, and LA Frohman. 3rd edition. McGraw-Hill 1995 p 289-383.
9. Robertson GL. Differential diagnosis of polyuria. Ann Rev Med 1988;39:425-442
10. Oelkers W. Adrenal insufficiency. NEJM 1996;335(16):1206-1212.
11. Dexter R. Hypopituitarism. In: Principles and Practice of Endocrinology and Metabolism. Ed. K. Becker. 2nd edition. JB Lippincott Co., Philadelphia. 1995:169-180.
12. Krishna A, Phillips L. Management of acromegaly: A review. Am J Med Sci 1994;308(6):370-375.
13. Aron DC, Tyrrell JB, Wilson CB. Pituitary tumors - Current concepts in diagnosis and management. West J Med 1995;162:340-352.
14. Samuels M, Ridgway EC. Glycoprotein-secreting pituitary adenomas. Bailliere's Clin Endo and Metab 1995;9(2):337-358.
15. Burke CW. The pituitary megatest: Outdated? Clin Endo 1992;36:133-134.
16. Rasmuson S., Olsson T., Hagg E. A low dose ACTH test to assess the function of the hypothalamic-pituitary-adrenal axis. Clin Endo 1996, 44, 151-156.
17. Clayton R.N., Short Shnacthen test versus insulin stress test for assessment of the hypothalmo-pituitary-adrenal axis. Clin Endo 1996, 44, 147-149.

2
Thyroid Disease

CAROLYN S. FELDKAMP, PHD & M. SAEED ZAFAR, MD

Physiology of the Thyroid-Pituitary-Hypothalamic Axis

The thyroid gland synthesizes the two hormones, thyroxine (T4) and 3,5,3'-triiodothyronine (T3). The thyroid cells extract iodine from the circulation. In the thyroid cells, the iodine is oxidized in the presence of H_2O_2 and thyroid peroxidase and immediately bound to thyroglobulin. This iodinated protein moves to the apex of the thyroid cell where tyrosine is iodinated into mono- and diiodotyrosine. At the apex of the thyroid cell, the monoiodotyrosine and diiodotyrosine molecules are coupled to form T3 and T4, respectively. The synthesis of T4 and T3 takes place on the surface of thyroglobulin. These hormones are then stored in the lumen of the thyroid follicle. During secretion, the intrafollicular contents are incorporated by endocytosis, then hydrolyzed and T4, T3, and thyroglobulin molecules are secreted into circulation. All these processes (the uptake of iodine, oxidation, hormone synthesis, and secretion of the thyroid hormones) are stimulated by thyroid stimulating hormone (TSH) (Fig.1).

Peripheral tissues, particularly liver and kidney, play an important role in storage, metabolism, and production of active thyroid hormone (T3). In these organs an enzyme, deiodinase, acts to convert T4 to T3. Eighty percent of T3 in circulation is derived through this peripheral mecha-

FIGURE 1. HYPOTHALAMIC-PITUITARY-THYROID AXIS

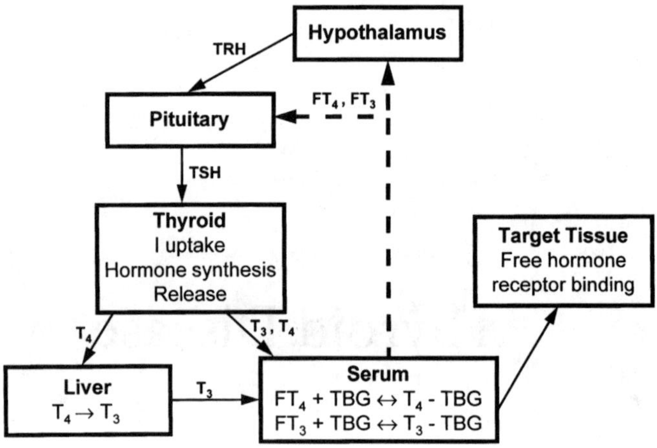

nism while the rest of the T3 is secreted directly from the thyroid gland. The liver also synthesizes three proteins which bind thyroid hormones in circulation: thyroid-binding globulin (TBG), transthyretin (TTR, previously called thyroid-binding pre-albumin), and albumin. In addition to intrathyroidal stores, the extrathyroidal tissues also store thyroid hormone with a volume of distribution of about 10 liters.

Thyroid hormones circulate in blood as bound and free forms. Normally, 0.02% of T4 and 0.3% of T3 are free. A dynamic equilibrium exists in circulation between these two forms. The tissue activity of the thyroid hormone is provided chiefly by the free hormones, although some bound thyroid hormone is also available to tissues for utilization. In most of the tissues, the circulating free T3 (FT3) is responsible for the biological effect of the thyroid hormone. Some tissues, however, utilize circulating T4 as well. The circulating free T4 (FT4) is converted in the pituitary and probably brain tissues by local deiodinase type II into intracellular T3. This T3 produced within the cells augments the biological effect of the FT3 derived from circulation.

The cellular effects of the thyroid hormones are produced through T3 receptors. Two types of thyroid hormone receptors (TR) have been identified, each with two isoforms: TR alpha-I and TR alpha-II, and TR beta-I and TR beta-II. While alpha I and the beta isoforms are utilized by T3 to produce the thyroid hormone effect, the alpha II isoform may antagonize the T3 function. The T3 receptor is unique in the super-family in that it remains attached to chromatin in the absence of T3 and inhibits the transcription of genes stimulated by T3. While in most of the tissues, the ligand-bound receptor bound to thyroid hormone response elements (TRE) increases the transcription of T3-responsive genes in the pituitary gland, T3-bound receptor bound to TRE will suppress the production of TSH.

Roughly 90 micrograms of T4 (120 mmol), 30 micrograms of T3, and 47-50 mmol of reverse T3 (rT3, 3,3',5'-triiodothyronine) are produced daily. Both the thyroid gland and extra thyroidal tissues are involved in T3 formation. The secretion of the daily amounts of hormones by the thyroid is fairly constant and is stimulated by the hypothalamic-pituitary axis, but inhibited by circulating FT4 and FT3. TSH is secreted episodically. The hypothalamic hormone thyrotropin-releasing hormone (TRH) stimulates the synthesis and secretion of TSH by the pituitary gland. Hypothalamic peptide, somatostatin, and amine (dopamine) dampen the secretion of TSH. Environmental influences can also affect the hypothalamic-pituitary axis. For example, the exposure to cold immediately after birth results in a sudden rise in TSH secretion. The hypothalamic-pituitary axis attempts to maintain a constant supply of thyroid hormones to peripheral tissues. The circulating free thyroid hormones T4 and T3 exercise an inhibitory influence on the secretion of TSH and TRH. Thus, a regulated hypothalamic-pituitary-thyroid-peripheral tissue axis maintains a fairly constant circulating free thyroid hormone blood level. When the free hormone levels decline, the TSH increases, acting to normalize the circulating FT4 and FT3 levels. On the other hand, when the FT4 and FT3 levels increase, the TSH secretion is inhibited.

Metabolism

Thyroid hormones are metabolized by a number of processes including deiodination, sulfation, conjugation and side chain cleavage. The major route of metabolism is through deiodination. T4 is metabolized chiefly by deiodinases that remove iodine atoms sequentially. Ultimately, thyronine with no iodine atoms is produced . The removal of iodine from the outer ring as the first step produces T3, the active hormone. The enzyme deiodinase I is present in the liver and kidney. It has an active site for selenium and at pH 6.5 to 7.5 removes the iodine from the outer ring producing T3. A similar enzyme present in the brain (deiodinase II) also produces T3 by removing iodine from the outer ring. It does not require selenium for its activity and is active at pH 6.5-7.5. It produces T3 in the brain and pituitary gland. The inner ring deiodination by deiodinase I at pH 8.0 to 8.5 and by deiodinase III (skin, brain, and placenta) produces rT3 which is inactive. The subsequent deiodination of the T3 and rT3 produces inactive molecules. The production of T3 by deiodinase I can be decreased in diseases of the liver and kidney, systemic diseases, as well as by certain drugs.

Aging and circulating thyroid hormones

Normal diurnal rhythm is established by four weeks after birth. Circulating T4 and T3 levels tend to be high during the first week after birth and then gradually decline to adult levels by 10-19 years of age. Thereafter, the levels of circulating thyroid hormones do not change.

Pregnancy and the thyroid economy

Pregnancy is a physiological state that affects the relationship among thyroid hormones in a complex, but predictable, fashion (Fig. 2). In the early part of pregnancy, the chorionic gonadotropin (HCG) produced by the placenta promotes the production of thyroid hormone by stimulating the thyroid gland, that is, HCG has a TSH-like effect. Also during this time, thyroid hormone binding proteins increase in circulation. Both of these changes increase the levels of bound thyroid hormones. If the increased binding capacity of the binding proteins is unable to absorb the added thyroid hormone produced by the thyroid as a result of HCG stimulation, the free thyroid hormone levels also will tend to rise. This tendency of free thyroid hormone levels to rise is dampened by a balancing downward shift in the TSH levels. Thus, in the early part of pregnancy, circulating thyroid hormone levels (bound T4 and T3) increase both due to increased amount of binding proteins as well as an increase in thyroid hormone produced by the TSH-like effect of HCG. Regulatory mechanisms react to these alterations in an attempt to keep free hormone levels normal. If the hormonal secretion from the thyroid gland exceeds the increased binding capacity of the binding proteins, FT4 levels will tend to increase and TSH will tend to shift downwards. On the other hand, if the binding capacity of proteins is greater than the hormone production increased by the TSH-like effect of HCG, the tendency for free hormone levels to decline will be reflected in an upward shift of the TSH levels in blood.

When in the later part of pregnancy (2nd and 3rd trimesters) the HCG levels decline, the TSH blood levels which had shifted downward in the early part of pregnancy return to the original levels. After delivery, the concentrations of binding proteins drop and a reversal of these processes occurs.

FIGURE 2. PATTERNS OF HORMONE CONCENTRATIONS DURING NORMAL PREGNANCY.

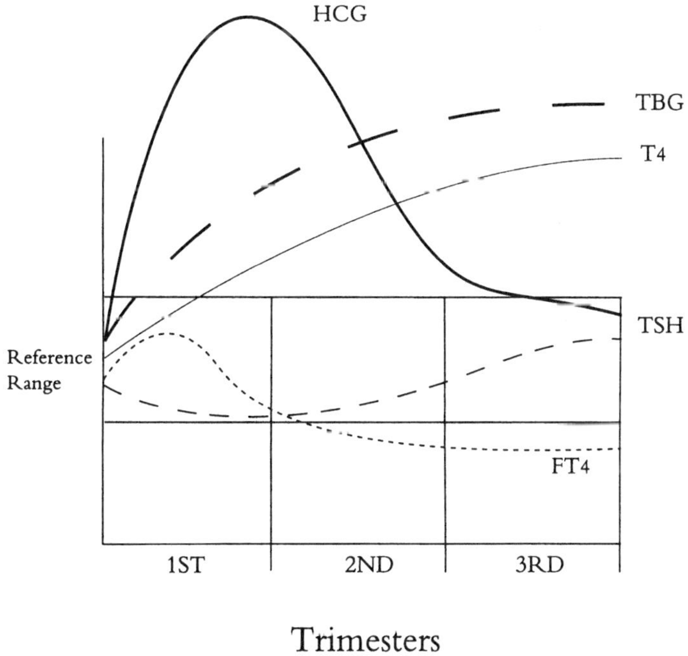

Adapted with permission from Fig 1 in Ref 2.

ALTERATIONS IN THYROID HORMONE ECONOMY IN NON-THYROIDAL DISEASE STATES

The extra thyroidal tissues, particularly liver and kidney, affect the thyroid economy by production of active hormone (T3), as well as by T4 and T3 metabolism into inactive products. The liver also is a major site of extra-thyroidal stores of thyroid hormones. Additionally, it produces the proteins that bind the thyroid hormones in circulation. It is, therefore, no surprise that diseases of liver and kidney, in particular, as well as systemic disorders affect thyroid hormone economy and circulating thyroid hormone blood levels. Theoretically, these alterations may be produced by one or more of the following mechanisms: 1) decreased activity of 5'-deiodinase producing less T3, 2) alteration in binding proteins, 3) altered metabolism of thyroid hormones, 4) interference with binding of T4 and T3 to binding proteins in circulation, 5) compensation by the hypothalamic-pituitary-thyroid axis to the above changes, 6) influence of drugs and various tissue factors on hypothalamic-pituitary-thyroid-peripheral tissue axis, and 7) perhaps others.

The alterations in the thyroid hormone economy in acute illness are complex. Neither the mechanism nor the significance of these alterations is completely understood. Furthermore, it is unknown if the administration of exogenous hormone is beneficial to the recovery of the individual. Some studies in adults and children suggest that treatment of hypothyroxinemia in severe non-thyroidal illness with T4 is not effective.

The levels of circulating thyroid hormones can be confusing. Generally, early in acute illness, T3 levels decrease and rT3 levels increase. As the severity of the disease increases from mild to moderate and perhaps as interfering substances appear in circulation, the binding of the hormone to the binding proteins is diminished. The bound T4 levels decline while the FT4 levels tend to shift upwards (but remain in the normal range) and TSH levels shift downwards. In advanced illness, T4 levels decline sharply to very low values. Recovery is accompanied by reversal of these processes (Table 1).

Disease-specific Variation

Caloric Deprivation

Acute caloric deprivation lowers total and FT3 within the first 24 hours reaching a nadir in one to two weeks. rT3 increases during this period. Total T4 is unchanged. FT4 levels are normal or slightly increased. TSH, after a slight downward shift, returns to baseline within four days. These effects are reversed by as little as 50 grams of glucose or protein, but not by fat.

Hepatic Disorders

Patients with hepatic cirrhosis have low serum T3 levels due to decreased production. T4 levels are either normal or low (due to decreased albumin and TTR). Serum FT4 and FT3 are generally within the normal range. TSH levels are within normal limits but may occasionally be minimally elevated.

Increased T4 and T3 levels are seen in acute infectious hepatitis, chronic active hepatitis, and billiary cirrhosis. This increase is due to increased production and release of TBG.

Renal Failure

Patients with chronic renal failure have low T3, but normal rather than elevated rT3. T4 levels are low, but FT4 and TSH levels are normal. The

TABLE 1. ALTERATIONS IN THYROID-PITUITARY HORMONES BY THYROID DISEASE, PHYSIOLOGICAL STATES, AND NON-THYROIDAL DISEASE

CONDITION	TSH	T4	FT4	T3	FT3	TBG	rT3
Thyroid Disease							
Primary hyperthyroidism	↓	↑	↑	↑	↑	N	
Primary hypothyroidism	↑	↓	↓	↓	↓	N	
Pituitary failure	↑*,N, ↓	N, ↓	↓				
Thyroid hormone resistance	↑	↑	↑	↑	↑	N	
TSH-secreting tumor	↑	↑	↑	↑	↑	N	
Non-thyroidal Conditions							
Pregnancy							
1st trimester	L-N	↑	N, ↑	↑		↑	↑
2nd & 3rd trimester	N	↑	N, ↓	↑	_	↑	↑
Systemic illness							
early	N	N	N	↓	N	N, ↑	↑
late	↓	↓	N, ↓	↓	↓	↓	↑
Starvation	↓,N	N	N, ↑	↓	↓		↑
Hepatitis							
chronic active	N, ↑	N, ↑	N	↑	↓	↑	N
active infections	N	N, ↑	N	↑	↓	↑	↑
Renal disease	N	↓	N	↓	N	↓	↑
Psychiatric disease	N,↑	N,↑	N,↑	N, ↑		N	↑
AIDS							
early	N, ↑	↑	N	N	–	↑	N, ↓
late		↓		↓	–, ↓	↑↑	

*Biologically inactive

thyroid hormone blood levels in nephrotic syndrome are similar, although patients lose T4, T3, and TBG through the kidney.

AIDS and AIDS-Related Complex

The circulating thyroid hormone blood levels in patients infected with HIV virus are somewhat different from patients with other non-thyroidal illnesses. An unexplained rise in serum TBG produces high circulating T4 levels. FT4 is normal. T3 is also normal rather than decreased. rT3 is normal or low. The serum TBG levels continue to increase as the patient moves from an asymptomatic stage to AIDS-related complex and finally to AIDS. The serum TSH levels are normal or may be slightly high. Ultimately, circulating T4 and T3 levels decline signifying a preterminal stage.

Psychiatric Disorders

A minority of patients with acute psychiatric illnesses may have elevated T4, FT4, and FTI at the time of admission. Serum T3 levels are generally normal or minimally elevated. rT3 is increased. Serum TSH levels may be elevated. TSH response to TRH may be blunted. Rapid reversal of these parameters, however, takes place.

Helpful Clues to Distinguish Thyroid Disease from Non-Thyroidal Causes of Abnormal Hormone Levels

The authors have found the following clues helpful when confronted with thyroid parameters from a patient with non-thyroidal illness (NTI).

- In hyperthyroidism, TSH is below 0.04 mU/L and FT4 may be high-normal or high. This degree of TSH suppression is extremely unlikely in NTI alone.
- In moderate to severe primary hypothyroidism, TSH will be unquestionably high and FT4 low. Such a combination of TSH and FT4 levels is uncommon in NTI.
- Confusion arises when FT4 is low and TSH is either low-normal or TSH is minimally high. These combinations of parameters are compatible with either NTI, mild primary hypothyroidism, or pituitary disease. Free thyroid index (FTI), calculated from T4 and T3 resin uptake (RUR) may provide a clue. While T4 is low in NTI, primary hypothyroidism and pituitary disease, RUR is almost always elevated or at the upper limit of normal in NTI and is almost always low-normal or lower than normal in primary hypothyroidism and hypopituitarism. rT3 is rarely needed and is available in few laboratories. rT3 is high in NTI except in some liver disorders, renal failure, or HIV-related disorders and low in hypothyroidism.
- When faced with an ill patient with confusing thyroid hormone values that suggest the diagnosis of hypopituitarism, measurement of serum cortisol values may be of help. In severe illness, plasma cortisol levels are generally high. This assessment, how-

ever, cannot be accomplished if the patient is receiving exogenous glucocorticoids.

- Finally, assessment of antithyroid antibodies may provide a clue to the presence of autoimmune thyroid disease.
- Concomitant thyroid disease and non-thyroidal illness can confuse the picture. Occasionally, NTI will normalize thyroid indices and mask thyroid disease. The most common example is the normalization of minimally elevated TSH of mild primary hypothyroidism. Mildly elevated T4 and T3 levels of hyperthyroidism may also become normal with superimposed NTI.

Thyroid Disorders

Hyperthyroidism

Hyperthyroidism is a state in which the body is exposed to an excessive amount of thyroid hormone. Common causes include Graves' disease, toxic nodule, toxic multinodular goiter, and thyroiditis. Clinical hyperthyroidism can also be produced by ingestion of excessive amount of thyroid hormones, T4 or T3. Except for thyroiditis, the change from euthyroidism to a hyperthyroid state and progression of hyperthyroidism is usually a slow and gradual process (Table 2). In fully developed hyperthyroidism, TSH levels are below 0.04 mU/L and FT4 levels are elevated. However, both these parameters do not become abnormal simultaneously. Usually, TSH levels fall to less than 0.04 mU/L before FT4 levels exceed the normal range. The patient at this stage may be asymptomatic and a state of "subclinical hyperthyroidism" is said to exist. Additionally, in Plummer's disease and early Graves' disease, the T3 levels rise before the increase in T4. When the TSH is suppressed to less than 0.04 mU/L with elevated T3 levels and normal FT4 levels, the patient is said to have "T3

Table 2. Progressive changes in thyroid hormones in hyperthyroidism

HORMONE	SUBCLINICAL	INTERMEDIATE	CLINICAL DISEASE
TSH	Low	Suppressed	Suppressed
T4	N	N	High
T3	N	High	High
FT4	N	N	High

toxicosis". It is important to appreciate that TSH levels may decline below the population normal range before T4 or FT4 levels become elevated.

Iatrogenic hyperthyroidism

Iatrogenic hyperthyroidism can be produced when patients are treated with T4 or T3. When the hyperthyroidism is produced by exogenous administration of T3, the TSH levels as well as FT4 will be low. T3 levels will be elevated, but may not be tested unless the ingestion of T3 is known.

Hyperthyroidism in pregnancy

The diagnosis of hyperthyroidism during pregnancy can be a challenge because of the complicating effects of the pregnancy on thyroid hormone levels in blood. In normal pregnancy TSH-like effects of HCG may produce high FT4 and subnormal TSH levels when HCG levels are at or near peak. This stage should not be confused with a thyroid disease. As the HCG levels decline, the thyroid hormone levels (FT4 and TSH) tend to return to normal. If TSH levels are below 0.04 mU/L and FT4 levels are high, a state of hyperthyroidism either due to thyroid disease or abnormally high HCG levels (hyperemesis gravidarum, choriocarcinoma) exists.

Transient hyperthyroidism

Thyroiditis is an inflammatory disorder of the thyroid of viral or autoimmune etiology. Inflammation releases thyroid stores from the gland, followed by loss of function of thyroid cells. Ultimately, recovery and restoration of normal function take place. In thyroiditis a spectrum of thyroid indices may be observed. In the early phase, the inflammation of the thyroid releases the thyroid hormone stores into circulation. Elevation in thyroid hormone levels suppresses TSH. The combined effects of low TSH and inflammation of the thyroid stop the synthesis of new thyroid hormones by the damaged cells. With the passage of time, circulating thyroid hormone levels decline to normal and then further to levels below normal. The TSH levels then start to rise. If the cells have regained the capacity to synthesize thyroid hormones, production will resume and both free thyroid hormones, total thyroid hormones, and then TSH will return to normal in succession.

It is obvious that early in the course, FT4 levels will be normal or high and TSH below normal. With progression, TSH declines further as FT4 levels increase. This is followed by normal FT4 levels and low TSH levels, normal FT4 and normal TSH levels followed by low FT4 and high TSH levels, normal FT4 and high TSH levels with ultimate return to normal FT4 and TSH levels and euthyroidism. The time course of the disease varies. It may take as long as 6 months to a year for the disorder to complete the cycle. Continually changing thyroid hormone parameters are a clue to the underlying disorders.

The term "transient hyperthyroidism," although true, is not a comprehensive description of this disorder. The hyperthyroidism is followed in succession by a "transient euthyroid state", followed by "transient hypothyroidism", and followed usually by euthyroidism. This is the usual course of events, however, occasionally mild persistent hypothyroidism is the sequela. If the disorder is mild and the early hyperthyroid phase is missed, the underlying disorder may not be appreciated and continually changing thyroid hormone concentrations may be confounding.

High TSH with hyperthyroidism

TSH levels are almost always low in hyperthyroidism. Occasionally, a hyperthyroid state exists with a high TSH and high FT4 levels. TSH-secreting pituitary tumor and thyroid hormone resistance confined to the pituitary gland will produce such a picture. TSH response to TRH is particularly helpful to identify and to differentiate between the two disorders. In TSH-secreting pituitary tumor, the administration of exogenous TRH fails to significantly alter the elevated TSH levels observed prior to administration of TRH. This contrasts with the further increase in TSH observed in hyperthyroxinemia of thyroid hormone resistance. In thyroid hormone resistance due to receptor aberrations, the thyrotroph responds to a higher quantity than usual of free thyroid hormones in the negative feedback loop. As with the pituitary tumor, TSH and FT4 are both elevated or TSH may be within the normal range with FT4 elevated.

Hypothyroidism

Primary hypothyroidism

In primary hypothyroidism, as FT4 levels start to decline, TSH levels increase. In fully developed hypothyroidism, FT4 values are low and TSH levels abundantly high. As in early hyperthyroidism, patients frequently pass through a stage of subclinical, or "compensated" hypothyroidism when FT4 levels are normal and TSH is minimally elevated (Table 3).

TABLE 3. PROGRESSIVE CHANGES IN THYROID HORMONES IN HYPOTHYROIDISM

TEST	MILD/SUBCLINICAL	MODERATE	CLINICAL
TSH	Elevated	High	High
T4	N	Low	Low
T3	N	N	Low
FT4	N	Low	Low

Central hypothyroidism

In central hypothyroidism, effective TSH stimulation of thyroid is diminished. TSH and FT4 levels are expected to be low. This occurs in advanced and total pituitary failure or, rarely, in hypothalamic dysfunction. Hypopituitarism is usually partial. FT4 levels may be accompanied by low, normal, or even high (minimal increase) TSH levels. The inappropriate TSH levels result from the measurement of biologically inactive TSH molecules.

Hypothyroidism following radioactive iodine (RAI) therapy

After RAI therapy for hyperthyroidism, FT4 levels decline before suppressed TSH levels return to normal. At this stage, FT4 and TSH levels are below normal and may be confused with central hypothyroidism. The patient may be clinically euthyroid or even complain of symptoms of hypothyroidism. If left untreated, and if the failure of the thyroid gland is progressive, TSH levels will ultimately rise above normal.

Treated hypothyroidism

Circulating thyroid hormone levels in patients treated with exogenous thyroid hormone depend on the agent used. If levothyroxine is used to attain euthyroidism, both FT4 and TSH levels are within the normal range. If T3 (cytomel) is used to bring TSH into the normal range, FT4 levels will be low but T3 levels are high.

Neonatal hypothyroidism

In primary neonatal or juvenile hypothyroidism TSH levels are elevated while T4, T3, and FT4 levels are low or low-normal for age. In central hypothyroidism, all thyroid hormones related measurements are low.

Effects of Binding Protein Aberrations on Thyroid Function Tests

- In addition to diseases of the liver, the capacity of thyroid hormone binding proteins may be abnormal either due to inherited abnormal levels of binding proteins, or due to increased affinity for binding hormones. When TBG concentration is low, the resulting low T4 concentration may be confused with hypothyroidism. However RUR is high, pointing to binding protein deficiency. Similarly, when TBG is high, circulating T4 is high, but RUR is low. Thankfully, FT4 and TSH levels are normal in this circumstance.
- An inherited abnormality of thyroid hormone binding by albumin which binds T4 with increased affinity will produce high T4 levels (dysalbuminemic hyperthyroxinemia). T3 levels are normal. RUR is not low in this condition since this test does not measure TTR. Thus, RUR is normal and FTI is high. TSH and FT4 are both normal and the patient is euthyroid.
- Rarely, in autoimmune disorders of the thyroid, patients may develop antibodies to T4 and/or T3. In such circumstances, T4 and/or T3 levels are elevated, with RUR changed in the opposing direction providing a clue to binding protein problems. If such individuals are hypothyroid and receiving hormone supplements, confusion may arise. Because of increased protein binding capacity for thyroid hormones, FT4 will decrease and TSH will increase. An increase in the dose of exogenous thyroid hormone becomes necessary.

Screening for Subclinical Thyroid Disease

Who should be tested beyond those with clinical suspicion of thyroid disease? The previous discussion related to the interpretation of hormone levels obtained in patients with thyroidal or non-thyroidal illness. However, there is no consensus for testing asymptomatic populations. Most groups do not recommend screening asymptomatic populations. The fo cus has been the detection of overt disease in the general, un-screened population. A pragmatic substitute for routine screening is the "recommendation for clinicians to maintain a low threshold for suspecting hypothyroidism...and to reserve testing for these patients."

The American College of Physicians has published clinical guidelines for screening for thyroid disease which take into account published data on prevalence, risk for complications, and appropriateness of treatment of subclinical disease. They recommend screening women older than 50 years of age for unsuspected, but symptomatic thyroid disease using sensitive TSH. Free T4 should be done if TSH is undetectable or >10 mU/L. Patients discovered by this screening protocol to have overt hypothyroidism (TSH > 10 mU/L and low FT4) or overt hyperthyroidism (TSH undetectable and high FT4) are likely to benefit from treatment. *Subclinical hyperthyroidism* and *subclinical hypothyroidism* as defined by these guidelines are patients whose TSH is undetectable, or > 10 mU/L, but who have normal FT4. Data were not sufficient for this group to recommend treatment of subclinical disease. However, this remains controversial and awaits more definitive studies. In the target screening population, patients with normal TSH should be screened every 2-5 years.

Some authors recommend routine testing of "high risk" populations including:

- neonates
- those with a higher prevalence of disease such as individuals > 60 years
- women
- those with dyslipidemia
- those with a family history
- those taking drugs which affect thyroid function e.g., lithium, amiodorone

Populations not recommended for screening include asymptomatic adults <35 years of age and acutely ill patients unless there is a strong suspicion that thyroid disease is contributing to the current illness.

The association of subclinical hypothyroidism with future progression to overt hypothyroidism, hypercholesterolemia and associated risk for cardiovascular disease, as well as the availablility of effective treatment, stimulated an analysis of the cost effectiveness of periodic screening for subclinical hypothyroidism by Danese, et al. TSH and cholesterol were included in a health examination every 5 years beginning at age 35. Their model suggests that the screening for hypothyroidism is favorable, especially in older women, and is cost-effective. No clinical experience with this approach has yet been reported.

Laboratory Tests Used in the Assessment of Thyroid Function: Normal Ranges, Sensitivity, Specificity, Problems with Interpretation

TSH (thyrotropin, thyroid stimulating hormone)

TSH plays a central role in the regulation of the thyroid economy. As illustrated in Fig 1, TSH and FT4 are inversely related. This relationship is log-linear, a 2-fold change in FT4 causing a 50-fold change in TSH. Thus, TSH is the earliest hormone to respond to changes in thyroid gland function and it is not uncommon to observe TSH outside the normal range while the FT4 is within the population normal range. Conversely, with certain exceptions such as pituitary disease, a normal TSH level is consistent with the euthyroid state. This has led some to use a TSH-first strategy in the evaluation of a patient for possible thyroid disease. Use of an algorithm that includes FT4 <u>only</u> when TSH is outside the normal range provides cost effective and appropriate thyroid testing in most settings, provided the algorithm is used in individuals with a normal pituitary gland (Fig 3). Interpretation of TSH and FT4 levels must take into account the physiological conditions and drugs that can affect TSH concentrations (Table 1 and Table 4).

Figure 3. Thyroid Testing Algorithm

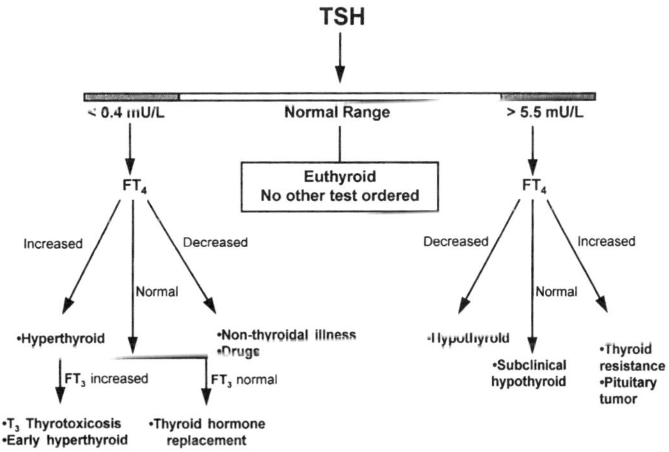

Designed for the initial evaluation of suspected thyroid disease. TSH is tested first. If TSH > 5.5 mU/L < 0.04 mU/L, free T4 (FT4) is run on the same specimen. Additional follow-up tests may be ordered, depending on the test results, clinical history, drug therapy, and concurrent illness. Not applicable for patients with suspected pituitary disease.

Sensitivity

Functional sensitivity is defined as the lowest concentration with a coefficient of variation (CV) of < or equal to 20%. Sensitivity of 0.01-0.05 mU/L achieved by most immunometric assays is adequate to clearly differentiate between fully developed hyperthyroidism (<0.04 mU/L) and euthyroidism.

Analytical Specificity/Interferences

TSH measurements are not affected by variations in thyroid binding proteins. Antibodies to various animal species (for example, human anti-mouse antibody, HAMA) can interfere with TSH assays by binding the animal antibodies used as reagents in the test. Prior exposure of the patient to animals or therapy with mouse monoclonal anti-tumor antibodies can cause false elevations in TSH levels.

TABLE 4. EFFECTS OF DRUG THERAPY ON THYROID HORMONE TESTS.

Drug	Notes	Binding Proteins	TSH	T4	T3	RUR	FT4
Glucocorticoids	T4 to T3 conversion decreased, Effects on binding proteins		N, ↓	↓	↓	↑	-
Dopamine	Effects on pituitary secretion		↓				
Lithium	Hypothyroidism in 5-10%		N,↑	N, ↓	N, ↓	N, ↓	N, ↓
Interferon-alpha	Exacerbates hypothyroidism		↑	↓	↓		↓
Interleukin-2	Exacerbates hypothyroidism		↑	↓	↓		↓
Iapanoic Acid	T4 to T3 dec.; Release inhibited		↑	↑	↓		N, ↑
Amiodarone	Inhibits deiodinase Cytotoxic to thyroid	↓	↑	N, ↑	↑	↑	
Testosterone	Decreases thyroid binding proteins	↓	N	↓	↓	↑	N
Estrogens	Increases thyroid binding proteins	↑	N	↑	↑	↓	N
Asparaginase			N	↓	↓	↑	
Phenytoin	Displaces T4 from TBG	N	N	↓	↓		N
Phenobarbital	Displaces T4 from TBG	N				N, ↑	
Heparin	Releases T4 from TBG *in vitro*	N	N	↓	N	N, ↑	N
Cholestyramine			N,↑	↓	N,		N
Clofibrate			N	↓	N, ↑		N
Carbamazepine	Displaces T4 from TBG	N		↓			
Colestipol			↑	↑	↓		

Up arrow = increases, down arrow = decreases, N = no significant change, remains in the normal range. Blank = not relevant or not typically measured in this condition.

Normal Range

Adult: 0.3-5.0 mU/L (may vary slightly with assay method).

Pediatric: Cord blood, <50 mU/L (variable, time dependent)

>1 month, same as adult range

TRH Test, (thyrotropin releasing hormone test).

The TRH test consists of measurements of TSH before and after administration of TRH. Administration of exogenous TRH normally elicits a rise in TSH concentration which reaches a peak at around 15-20 minutes and returns to baseline in 60 minutes. (The extent of rise depends on the dose of TRH used.) Normal elderly men may have initially low-normal TSH levels and a somewhat blunted rise in serum TSH after TRH administration. In primary hyperthyroidism, the TSH levels are low and fail to rise further after TRH administration. In primary hypothyroidism TSH levels are elevated and rise briskly after TRH administration. In hypothalamic-pituitary disease the pattern of response is altered; the peak rise is blunted, delayed, and returns to baseline after 60 minutes. With the availability of sensitive TSH, this test has been abandoned for most evaluations of hyperthyroidism, but it is still useful in TSH-secreting pituitary tumors and thyroid hormone resistance.

Free Thyroxine (FT4)

In serum, free hormones are in equilibrium with hormone bound to binding proteins. Though most FT4 methods accurately distinguish hyperthyroidism and hypothyroidism from euthyroidism., levels are best interpreted in conjunction with TSH. Physiological concentrations of FT4 may be affected by a variety of drugs, non-thyroidal diseases, pituitary disease, and normal physiological conditions such as pregnancy (Table 1).

Influence of Methods of Analysis on Test Results

- FT4 measured by equilibrium dialysis is the "gold standard," but the method is slow, labor intensive and not suitable for routine evaluations. It is used only for research or very unusual cases.
- FT4 measured by immunoassay. A variety of formats including a one-step, analog tracer format or a 2-step, sequential assay format are available on many automated instruments.

Interferences/ Considerations for Interpretation of Results.

Most contemporary immunoassays minimize interferences from varying concentrations of binding proteins in the patient sample.

Normal Range

Adult: 0.89-1.9 ng/dL (varies slightly with method). 2nd and 3rd trimester pregnancy: 0.65-1.2 ng/dL.

Thyroxine (T4)

T4 is the thyroid hormone circulating in highest concentration. T4 (free and protein-bound) is measured by competitive immunoassays that are generally reliable. Since circulating concentrations are influenced by binding proteins and a variety of clinical conditions and drugs, the test has been largely replaced by FT4 or FTI (Table 1).

Normal Range

Adult: 4.6-11.6 ug/dL (varies slightly with method). Pediatric: Cord blood, 6.6-17.5 μg/dL. After 1 month, same as adult range.

Resin Uptake Ratio (RUR)

RUR, also called T3 Resin Uptake, is used to assess whether alterations in total T4 are the result of increased or decreased binding proteins or due to alterations in thyroid function (Fig 4). RUR is inversely proportional to unsaturated thyroid hormone binding sites, predominately TBG, and is expressed as a ratio of the patient response to the normal response. RUR decreases (RUR$<$1) when binding proteins increase (for example, in pregnancy) or are relatively unsaturated with bound T4 as in hypothyroidism. RUR increases (RUR$>$1) when binding proteins decrease from normal or are relatively saturated with bound T4 as in hyperthyroidism. RUR is used in conjunction with T4 to calculate FTI.

A number of variations of 'uptake' tests are commercially available, all of which provide a measure of the effect of thyroid hormone binding proteins. The normal ranges and the calculations of FTI may vary with the individual laboratory.

Normal Range

RUR, adult: 0.8-1.2

FIGURE 4. PROCEDURE AND INTERPRETATION OF RESIN UPTAKE RATIO TEST (A.K.A. T3-RESIN UPTAKE OR RESIN UPTAKE)

$$T3^* + TBG_{unsat} \leftrightarrow T3^*\text{-}TBG$$

Procedure:

1) Incubate patient sample or normal control (containing TBG) with labeled T3 (T3*).

2) Add resin to "take up" remaining unbound T3*.

3) Measure T3* uptake in patient and normal control.

4) Calculate Resin Uptake Ratio (RUR) = T3*-uptake in patient/ T3*-uptake in normal control.

Interpretation:

- T3*-uptake is inversely proportional to unsaturated TBG (TBG_{unsat}).
- RUR ≈ 1 when patient is normal. (Normal range = 0.8-1.2)
- RUR > 1 when patient TBG is saturated relative to normal control (primary hyperthyroid).
- RUR < 1 when TBG concentration is increased (e.g., estrogens).
- RUR < 1 when TBG is unsaturated relative to normal control (primary hypothyroid).
- RUR > 1 when TBG concentration is decreased.

Free Thyroxine Index (FTI)

This index is calculated as Total T4 x Resin Uptake Ratio (RUR). This index is proportional to FT4. FTI correlates well with FT4 and inversely with TSH and is an acceptable substitute for free thyroid hormone measurement in most populations. In some cases, such as severe non-thyroidal illness, RUR does not fully compensate and does not adjust the T4 into the normal range. Since measured FT4 may be low in NTI, simply the elevated RUR may provide a clue to the mechanism of the low T4 and low FT4 observed in these conditions. In the evaluation of some complex or ambiguous cases, some endocrinologists still prefer to see separately the measurement of total T4 and the RUR as an independent measure of binding proteins.

Normal Range

FTI, adult: 5.5-10.0 ug/dL (varies slightly with method).

Note that the units of FTI are the same as total T4. The normal range of FTI, calculated individually from normal subjects, is somewhat more narrow than the T4 population normal range. This observation supports the hypothesis that individuals have an individual pituitary 'set-point', or narrow range for free thyroid hormones at which point TSH begins to respond.

Interpretation

- Hyperthyroid. RUR is >1; T4 is elevated. Thus, FTI (T4 x RUR) is elevated and FTI is >T4, confirming the hyperthyroid state.
- Hypothyroid. RUR is <1; T4 is low. Thus, FTI is relatively decreased and FTI is <T4, accentuating the impression of hypothyroidism.
- Euthyroid. Increased or decreased binding proteins result in elevated or decreased total T4 concentration. RUR changes will be opposite of T4. Thus, FTI will move toward the middle of the normal range, confirming euthyroidism. For example, in pregnancy TBG increases, resulting in increased T4. In this condition RUR is <1. FTI will be <T4 (that is, T4 x a factor <1). RUR "normalizes" T4.

FTI correlates with FT4 and is an acceptable estimate of free thyroid hormone in most populations. In some cases, such as severe non-thyroidal illness, RUR does not fully compensate and does not adjust the T4 into the normal range. Since measured FT4 also may be low in NTI, the observation of an elevated RUR may provide a clue to the mechanism of low T4 and low FT4.

Triiodothyronine (T3)

T3 in blood is derived predominantly from peripheral conversion (deiodination) of T4. Thyroid secretion contributes only up to 20% in normal circumstances. The contribution of the thyroid to circulating T3 increases, however, in states of thyroid overactivity. Like T4, T3 circulates predominantly bound to thyroid binding proteins, TBG, albumin, and prealbumin. T3 reflects the hormone stores in blood. Like T4, the T3 levels are high in fully developed hyperthyroidism. However, in very early hyperthyroidism T3 concentrations are high while T4 levels are still normal.

The main clinical utility of the test is to confirm early hyperthyroidism when TSH is low, but FT4 is in the normal range (T3 thyrotoxicosis). The test is not needed to confirm advanced hyperthyroidism with suppressed TSH and elevated FT4. The test is also *not necessary* in the diagnosis of hypothyroidism.

Normal Range

80-200 ng/dL (varies slightly with method).

Free T3

FT3 is the bioactive thyroid hormone and is measured independent of binding proteins by equilibrium dialysis and, more commonly, analog-tracer competitive binding immunoassay. Because of the analytical difficulties relating to the very low concentration of FT3 in serum, FT4 is the more reliable and preferred test to assess thyroid function. FT3 is useful to confirm early hyperthyroidism in a patient with altered binding proteins (estrogens) and who has suppressed TSH, but normal FT4, that is, T3 thyrotoxicosis, a rare condition. Because of the influence of binding proteins and drugs on total T3 concentrations (similar to T4), FT3 is preferred over T3.

Normal Range

Adult: 200-500 pg/dL (varies slightly with method).

Reverse T3 (rT3)

rT3 is elevated in severe non-thyroidal illness. Theoretically rT3 could help differentiate between the low FT4 levels of systemic disease from the low FT4 levels due to thyroid or pituitary failure. However, TSH serves this purpose in most circumstances (high in hypothyroidism, low or normal in severe illness).

In newborns with suspiciously high TSH and concomitant severe illness, early diagnosis and treatment of hypothyroidism are essential. The situation may be confusing since newborns normally have high TSH which varies with age. An elevated rT3 may clarify the diagnosis by confirming the impact of the illness on thyroid hormones. rT3 has also been reported to be elevated in anorexia nervosa, but is rarely needed since an elevated cortisol is a signal of anorexia nervosa. The measurement is not available in most laboratories and *usually is not necessary.*

Thyroglobulin (TG)

Thyroglogulin is the thyroid protein on which thyroid hormones are synthesized. Serum concentrations of TG are generally proportional to thyroid mass and increase with tissue damage or increased thyroid activity. Although TG is not a tumor marker, it is useful in following the course of patients with treated thyroid carcinoma. In a patient who has been treated for differentiated thyroid carcinoma, TG should be almost non-detectable. Increasing serum levels of TG suggests persistence or growth of thyroid cancer.

Analytical Methods

TG is measured by immunoassays in various formats all of which suffer from lack of sensitivity and variable analytical specificity. Use of an international reference preparation (Community Bureau of Reference (CBR) of the Commission of the European Communities) is hoped to improve inter-method comparison. Interference in TG assays may occur when patients' sera contain antibodies to TG. High dose "hook" effects have been reported (inappropriately low results measured in patients whose actual concentration is very high).

Normal Range

Normal range depends on the assay method and sensitivity of the assay. Serial samples using the same method over a period of time is the preferred application of this test.

Thyroid Autoantibodies

Several diseases of the thyroid gland such as Graves' disease, Hashimoto's disease, and postpartum thyroiditis are caused by autoimmune processes. These conditions are associated with one or more antibodies to various proteins of the thyroid gland, including anti-TG, anti-thyroid peroxidase (anti-TPO, formerly thyroid microsomal antibody), and anti-TSH receptor (anti-TR). Anti-TR may act by either stimulating the TSH receptor, or blocking the receptor.

In spite of the association with autoimmune thyroid disease, thyroid antibodies offer little additional diagnostic value. Anti-TPO alone is recommended as a cost-effective and sensitive assessment of autoimmune etiology. The presence of anti-TPO has been used by some to support the diagnosis of autoimmune disease; however positive anti-TPO does not exclude the presence of malignancy. Anti-TG assayed in conjunction with the TG immunoassay is used to rule out potential assay interference. The recommended use of anti-TR is to assist in the diagnosis of Graves' disease in a pregnant patient or in the management of a pregnant patient with current or previous history of Graves' disease. The latter use is to assess the risk of fetal or neonatal thyrotoxicosis since some maternal anti-TR crosses the placenta.

Analytical Methods

Thyroid autoantibodies are detected by qualitative or quantitative immunoassays in varying formats. Results are reported as U/mL or as a titer. Unfortunately, results among methods vary widely because of different specificities of the antibodies, different, sometimes complex, antigens used to detect the antibodies, and a lack of consensus standards. Normal ranges are variable depending on the specificity and precision of the assay.

Utilization of Laboratory Tests in the Diagnosis and Monitoring of Thyroid Disease

Recommendations for Testing

For diagnosis and monitoring treatment of thyroid disease, either FT4 direct measurement or another estimate of free thyroxine such as FTI can be used. The choice depends primarily on availability and cost.

- A TSH-first algorithm which reflexes to FT4 is a medically efficient and cost effective initial evaluation for most suspected thyroid disease. *Do not use this algorithm to assess patients with possible pituitary disease.*
- To confirm the diagnosis of thyroid disease, FT4 is preferred over FT3.
- If T3-thyrotoxicosis is suspected (low TSH with normal FT4), FT3 is preferred over total T3, if available.
- Monitor thyroid hormone replacement therapy with TSH.
- Monitor suppression therapy for thyroid cancer with *sensitive* TSH.
- Follow thyroid ablation for hyperthyroidism with FT4.
- A TSH-first algorithm is effective to screen asymptomatic individuals in special or high risk populations, e.g., the elderly, women over 60 years of age, neonates, individuals taking drugs known to affect the thyroid, individuals with a personal or family history of thyroid disease.

Interpretive Hints when TSH and FT4 Results Seem Discrepant

- When TSH is low and FT4 normal: FT3 may confirm T3-thyrotoxicosis.
- TSH & FT4 both increased: Suspect thyroid resistance or pituitary tumor. (TSH may be in the upper normal range with FT4 increased in thyroid hormone resistance. This would not be apparent if an algorithm which reflexes only when TSH is abnor-

mal were used for initial testing.)

- TSH & FT4 both low-normal: NTI or suspect central hypothyroidism (hypothalamic or hypopituitary).
- TSH/T4 are hormones in dynamic equilibrium in each individual. In treated hypothyroidism, the blood levels may not reach steady-state for 4-6 weeks. Wait 8 weeks after thyroid hormone dose adjustment to assess the effect.
- In patients being treated with thyroid hormone replacement, low TSH with normal FT4 may suggest over-replacement.
- Consider patient compliance, change in drug formulation, drug absorption, and assay interference. Non-compliance is common.
- Consider the impact of drugs, systemic illness, or pregnancy in the interpretation of TSH and FT4 <u>before</u> initiating extensive follow-up or esoteric diagnoses.

Selected Reading

1. Brent G, Hershman J. Thyroxine therapy in patients with severe non-thyroidal illness and low serum thyroxine. J Clin Endocrinol Metab 1986; 63:1-8.
2. Burrow G, Fisher D, Larsen P. Maternal and fetal thyroid function. N Eng J Med 1994; 331(16):1072-1078.
3. Danese M, Powe N, Sawin C, Ladenson P. Screening for mild thyroid failure at the periodic health examination. A decision and cost-effectiveness analysis. JAMA 1996; 276(4):285-292.
4. Feldkamp C, Carey J. An algorithmic approach to thyroid function testing in a managed care setting. 3-year experience. Am J Clin Pathol 1996; 105:11-16.
5. Feldkamp C, Zafar M. Evaluation of thyroid status during pregnancy. Diag Endocrinol Metab 1997; 15(4):105-113.
6. Feldt-Rasmussen U. Analytical and clinical performance goals for testing autoantibodies to thyroperoxidase, thyroglobulin, and thyrotropin receptor. Clin Chem 1996; 42(1):160-163.
7. Fisher D. Maternal-fetal thyroid function in pregnancy. Clin Perinatol 1983; 10(3):615-626.
8. Lambert M, Zech F, DeNayer P, Jamez J, Vandercam B. Thyroxine-

binding globulin (but not cortisol-binding globulin and sex hormone-binding globulin) associated with the progression of human immunodeficiency virus infection. Amer J Med 1990; 89:748-751.

9. LoPresti J, Fried J, Spencer C, Nicoloff J. Unique alteration of thyroid hormone indices in the acquired immunodeficiency syndrome(AIDS). Ann Intern Med 1989; 110:970-975.

10. Sawin C, ed. Laboratory Support for the Diagnosis and Monitoring of Thyroid Disease. National Academy of Clinical Biochemistry, 1996:64. (Kaplan L, ed. Standards of Laboratory Practice

11. Spencer CA. Clinical utility and cost-effectiveness of sensitive thyrotropin assays in ambulatory and hospitalized patients. Mayo Clin Proc 1988; 63:1214-1222.

12. Spencer CA, Presti JSL, Patel A, Guttler RB, Eigen A, Shen D, Gray D, Nicoloff JT. Applications of a new chemiluminometric thyrotropin assay to subnormal measurement. J Clin Endocrinol Metab 1990; 70:453-460.

13. Styra R, Joffe R, Singer W. Hyperthyroxinemia in major affective disorders. Acta Psychiatr Scand 1991; 83:61-63.

14. Surks MI, Chopra IJ, Mariash CN, Nicoloff JT, Solomon DH. American Thyroid Association. Guidelines for use of laboratory tests in thyroid disorders. JAMA 1990; 263:1529-1532.

15. Vanderpump M, Ahlquist J, Franklyn J, Clayton R. Consensus statement for good practice and audit measures in the management of hypothyroidism and hyperthyroidism. Br Med J 1996; 313:539-544.

16. Wartofsky L, Burman K. Alterations in thyroid function in patients with systemic illness: the "euthyroid sick syndrome". Endocr Rev 1982; 3:164-217.

17. Weetman A. Hypothyroidism: screening and subclinical disease. Br Med J 1997; 314:1175-1178.

3
Laboratory Approaches to Diseases of the Adrenal Cortex & Adrenal Medulla

WILLIAM E. WINTER, MD

Introduction

The production of glucocorticoids and mineralocorticoids by the adrenal cortex is necessary for health. Either an excess or a deficiency of these hormones produces serious clinical disease. In the first two sections of this chapter, adrenocortical insufficiency and excess will, respectively, be discussed. In the last section of this chapter, pheochromocytoma, a neoplastic and hormonally active disease of the adrenal medulla, will be discussed.

I) Adrenocortical Insufficiency

The hormonal products of the adrenal cortex are mineralocorticoids (e.g., aldosterone from the zona glomerulosa), glucocorticoids (e.g., cortisol from the zona fasiculata), and adrenal sex steroids (e.g., the adrenal androgens dehydroepiandrosterone and androstenedione from the zona reticularis). Deficiencies or excesses of these hormones cause serious clinical disease. Cortisol stimulates glucose production through hepatic gluconeogenesis and inhibits the action of insulin at insulin target tissues. These metabolic effects raise blood glucose levels. Cortisol also helps to maintain lysosomal integrity in cells and maintains vascular tone (e.g., acting as an anti-stress or anti-shock hormone). Aldosterone functions to conserve sodium, and "waste" potassium and hydrogen ion via their excretion in the urine (Figure 1). The gonads and adrenal cortex share many metabolic pathways for steroid hormone biosynthesis (Figure 2).

FIGURE 1. REGULATION OF ALDOSTERONE SECRETION

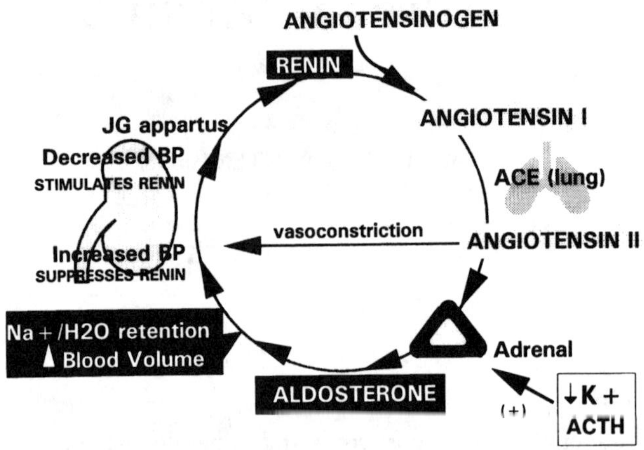

Renin is released by the juxtaglomerular apparatus in response to decreased renal perfusion from decreased cardiac output and/or decreased blood pressure. Renin cleaves renin-substrate (angiotensinogen) to angiotensin I. Angiotensin I is converted to angiotensin II in the lungs by angiotensin-converting enzyme (ACE). Angiotensin II is the body's most powerful endogenous vasoconstrictor. This directly acts to raise blood pressure via vasoconstriction. Angiotensin II acts on the zona glomerulosa of the adrenal cortex to release aldosterone. Aldosterone stimulates the distal convoluted tubule of the nephron to increase sodium absorption in exchange for potassium and hydrogen ion that are wasted into the urine. Increased sodium reabsorption leads to increased water reabsorption, increased circulating blood volume, and a rise in renal perfusion. If renal perfusion is adequately restored, renin secretion is suppressed in this negative feedback loop. Hypokalemia and adrenocorticotrophic hormone (ACTH) are both minor stimulators of aldosterone secretion. ACTH stimulates 11ß-hydroxylase which is expressed in the zona glomerulosa (not pictured). JG = juxtaglomerular; BP = blood pressure.

FIGURE 2. ADRENOCORTICAL STEROID HORMONE BIOSYNTHESIS

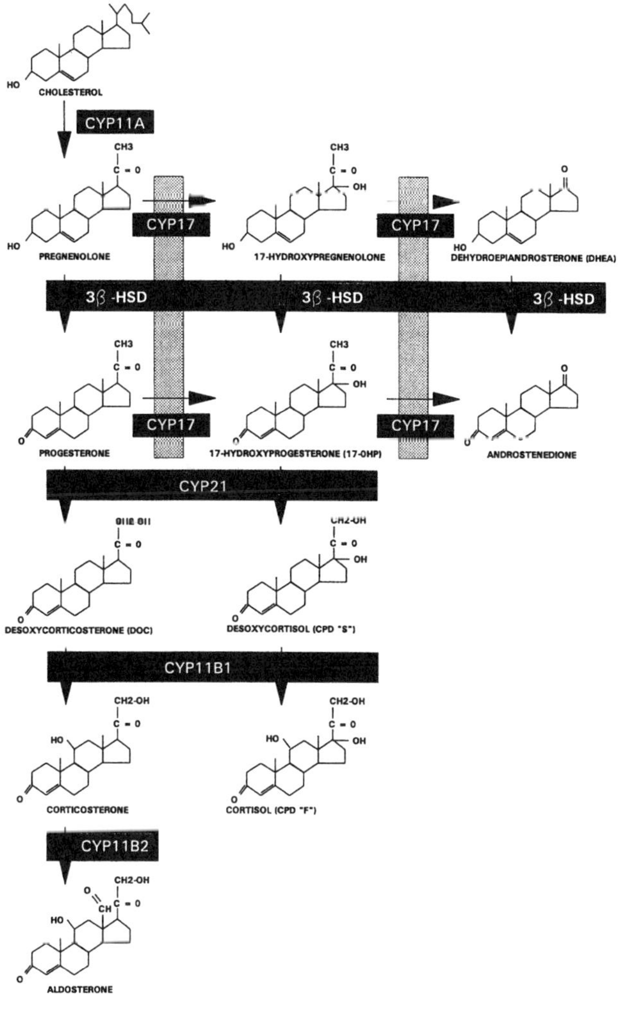

Cholesterol is converted to pregnanelone by the action of 20,22-lyase (desmolase) that is encoded by CYP11A. By the 17-hydroxylase activity of CYP17, pregnanelone is converted to 17-hydroxypregnanelone. By the 17,20 lyase (desmolase) activity of CYP17, 17-hydroxypregnanelone is converted to dehydroepiandrosterone. The only non-P450 enzyme, 3ß-hydroxysteroid dehydrogenase (sometimes abbreviated as 3ß-ol) converts pregnanelone to progesterone, 17-hydroxpregnanelone to 17-hydroxyprogesterone, and dehydroepiandrosterone to androstenedione. Likewise, by the 17-hydroxylase activity of CYP17, progesterone is converted to 17-hydroxyprogesterone (17-OHP). By the 17,20 lyase (desmolase) activity of CYP17, 17-hydroxyprogesterone is converted to androstenedione. In the gonad, androstenedione is the precursor of both testosterone and estradiol. In the zona glomerulosa, 21-hydroylase encoded by CYP21 converts progesterone to desoxycorticosterone (DOC). DOC is transformed into corticosterone by the action of 11ß-hydroxylase which is encoded by CYP11B1. Aldosterone is formed in two steps from corticosterone by the action of aldosterone synthase encoded by CYP11B2. In the zona fasciculata, 21-hydroxylase (CYP21) converts 17-hydroxyprogesterone to desoxycortisol. Desoxycortisol is transformed into cortisol by the action of 11ß-hydroxylase (CYP11B1). The formation of the adrenal androgens occurs in the zona reticularis.

A) Clinical Symptoms and Signs of Adrenocortical Insufficiency

Deficient cortisol production causes vascular instability, hypotension, and hypoglycemia, especially at times of severe stress. Patients feel weak with general malaise, loss of energy, and may display nausea, vomiting , or diarrhea. Primary adrenocortical failure is termed Addison disease after the 19th century English physician that described this condition. The clinical features of Addison disease include symptoms of weakness, lethargy/tiredness, increased fatigability, anorexia, nausea, vomiting, diarrhea (sometimes alternating with constipation), weight loss, abdominal pain, salt craving, muscle and joint pain, and postural dizziness. The signs of Addison disease encompass mottled skin pigmentation, increased pigmentation, decreased hair growth, hypotension, dehydration, tachycardia, and pallor. Laboratory findings in primary adrenal insufficiency include hypoglycemia, a normocytic normochromic anemia, modest eosinophilia, and relative lymphocytosis. Hyponatremia, hyperkalemia, hyperchloremia, decreased serum HCO_3^-, mild systemic acidosis, relatively alkaline urine (RTA type IV), and azotemia result from mineralocorticoid deficiency. Relative or absolute hyperchloremia may be masked by electrolyte depletion and hyponatremia. Psychiatric symptoms of organic brain syndrome (eg., impaired memory, confusion), depression, and psychosis may affect up to 40% of patients.

With primary adrenal insufficiency, hyperpigmentation results from elevated ACTH concentrations. In contrast, patients with secondary or tertiary adrenal insufficiency from, respectively, ACTH or CRH deficiency, do not exhibit hyperpigmentation. As well, patients deficient in ACTH or CRH do not manifest severe dehydration, hypotension, hyperkalemia, or acidosis because mineralocorticoids are not lacking in such circumstances. Signs and symptoms resulting from ACTH or CRH deficiency are usually mild compared to Addison disease (primary adrenocortical failure) and display hyponatremia but not hyperkalemia.

Inability to respond to acute stress precipitates "Addisonian crisis" where patients present with profound shock, hypotension, hypoglycemia, acidosis, hyponatremia, and hyperkalemia. Addisonian crisis is much more typical of primary adrenal failure than isolated ACTH deficiency. Untreated, Addisonian crisis can cause hypotension, vascular shock, and death.

B) Causes of Adrenocortical Insufficiency

Primary adrenocortical failure can be caused by autoimmunity, hemorrhage, infection (eg., tuberculosis), trauma, adrenalectomy, infiltrative disease, inborn errors of adrenocortical hormonogenesis (eg., congenital adrenal hyperplasia, see below), adrenoleukodystrophy, familial glucocorticoid deficiency, congenital adrenocortical hypoplasia, and certain drugs. Autoimmune destruction of the adrenal cortex is now the most common cause of primary adrenocortical failure. ACTH deficiency causing secondary adrenocortical insufficiency can result from suppression of the hypothalamic-pituitary-adrenal axis with exogenous glucocorticoids, destructive or compressive pituitary tumors and their treatment, hypothalamic tumors and their treatment (leading to CRH deficiency), cerebral trauma, irradiation, infection, bleeding, congenital malformations of the pituitary gland or hypothalamus, and idiopathic hypopituitarism.

Isolated mineralocorticoid deficiency is extremely rare. The most common cause of isolated mineralocorticoid deficiency is deficient renin production from renal disease due to interstitial nephropathy or diabetic nephropathy. Rarely aldosterone deficiency results from CYP11B2 deficiency. This enzyme is responsible for the conversion of corticosterone into aldosterone via a two step process of 18-hydroxylation followed by 18-oxidation. Patients with adrenocortical hypofunction usually experience cortisol deficiency or combined deficiencies of cortisol and aldosterone (eg., primary adrenocortical failure). Isolated cortisol deficiency results from ACTH (secondary adrenocortical insufficiency) or CRH deficiency (tertiary adrenocortical insufficiency). In patients with primary adrenocortical failure, glucocorticoid deficiency may precede mineralocorticoid deficiency (or rarely, vice versa).

C) Diagnostic Workup for Adrenocortical Insufficiency

Cortisol levels of <5 mg/dL in the AM or during times of stress are presumptive evidence of glucocorticoid (cortisol) deficiency. Levels ≥20 mg/dL essentially exclude cortisol deficiency. At times of crisis when Addison disease is suspected, the physician should draw cortisol levels and rapidly administer saline and glucocorticoids in pharmacologic doses (eg., 4 mg/M^2 of dexamethasone stat). The patient is treated for presumed Addisonian crisis until the next immunoassay run when the cortisol concentration is measured. *Stat cortisols are not required for patient management.* A sample for ACTH measurement can be stored by the laboratory if at a later time this measurement is desired.

The approach described below for the evaluation of suspected glucocorticoid deficiency is intended to provide a logical, step-by-step evaluation of adrenocortical function in an economically prudent and timely fashion (Figure 3). Patients with clinically suspected glucocorticoid deficiency are arranged into 4 groups dependent on clinical presentation, and their AM fasting or stress cortisol levels:

1) Patients presenting in acute Addisonian crisis.
2) Patients not acutely ill with abnormally low stress/AM cortisol levels <5mg/dL
3) Patients not acutely ill with potentially low stress/AM cortisol levels 5-<20mg/dL
4) Patients not acutely ill with normal stress/AM cortisol levels ≥20 mg/dL.

1) Patients Presenting with Addisonian Crisis

For the patient that arrives in the medical care facility with hypotension, hypoglycemia, hyperpigmentation, hyponatremia, hyperkalemia, and systemic acidosis that are otherwise unexplained, the diagnosis of Addison disease (primary adrenocortical failure) is strongly suggested. Confirmation of the diagnosis is afforded by a cortisol concentration of <5 mg/dL at this time of stress. An elevated plasma ACTH level at the time of acute stress in the face of a low cortisol level supports the diagnosis of Addison disease.

If further confirmation of the diagnosis of Addison disease is desired, the workup can proceed to a **One-hour ACTH Stimulation Test** or an **Insulin Tolerance Test** (ITT). In the **ITT**, hypoglycemia provides a powerful central stimulant to the release of CRH inducing ACTH and subsequent cortisol secretion (see chapter 1 for the **ITT** procedure). Some authors believe that the **ITT** is indicated only when recent ACTH or CRH deficiency is suspected and the **One-Hour ACTH Stimulation Test** could be falsely normal. Otherwise, the **One-Hour ACTH Stimulation Test** provides similar information to the ITT. In patients with a clinical history that suggests potential ACTH deficiency (eg., children following surgery for craniopharyngioma), the ITT can be performed to concurrently evaluate cortisol and growth hormone (GH) response to hypoglycemia. The **One-hour ACTH Stimulation Test** is much easier, safer, and cheaper to perform than the **ITT**. As neither of these tests differentiate primary adrenocortical failure from ACTH deficiency, a **Two-day ACTH Stimulation Test** can be performed instead. Despite prolonged stimulation from exogenous

FIGURE 3. GLUCORTICOID DEFICIENCY SUSPECTED ON CLINICAL GROUNDS

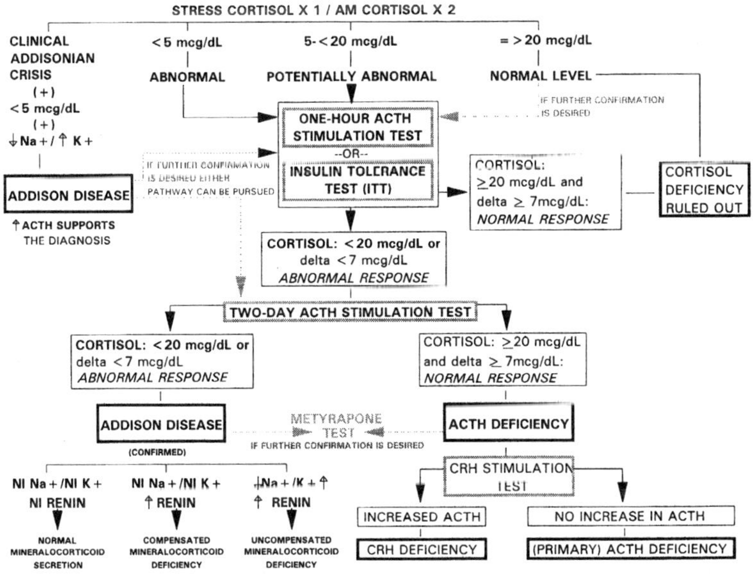

In patients who present in Addisonian crisis with supporting electrolyte changes and low cortisol, the diagnosis of Addison disease is established. In patients with suspected adrenocortical insufficiency , stress or AM cortisols ≥20 mg/dL virtually exclude glucocorticoid insufficiency. However, further testing can involve either a one-hour ACTH (cortrosyn) stimulation test or an insulin tolerance test. At least one of these tests is required in patients with suspected glucocorticoid insufficiency with stress or AM cortisol levels <20 mg/mL. After ACTH or insulin-induced hypoglycemia, cortisol levels ≥20 mg/dL with a change over baseline of ≥7 mg/dL rules out glucocorticoid insufficiency. Abnormal responses are consistent with glucocorticoid insufficiency. The two-day ACTH stimulation test is helpful in differentiating primary (Addison disease) from central (ACTH deficiency) adrenal insufficiency. With Addison disease, mineralocorticoid function must be evaluated by measuring electrolytes and renin. As well, aldosterone measurements may be necessary (not pictured). Although rarely pursued, the CRH stimulation test can assist in differentiating primary ACTH deficiency from CRH deficiency (secondary ACTH deficiency).

ACTH in the **Two-day ACTH Stimulation Test**, in Addison disease the cortisol levels remain <5 mg/dL confirming primary adrenocortical failure.

If a **One-hour ACTH Stimulation Test** , an **ITT**, or a **Two-day ACTH Stimulation Test** is to be performed, maintenance doses of dexamethasone should be provided. Dexamethasone is used because this glucocorticoid does not cross react in the cortisol immunoassay. Thus, any changes in cortisol concentration following stimulation will reflect endogenous production of cortisol.

2) Patients with Suspected Glucocorticoid Deficiency Who Do Not Present Acutely Ill

When a patient presents with signs or symptoms suggestive of (but not diagnostic for) glucocorticoid deficiency, *a laboratory investigation should be pursued before glucocorticoid replacement therapy is initiated.* If a patient is ill enough to require acute glucocorticoid therapy, they are evaluated similarly to patients with frank Addisonian crisis.

Fasting cortisol levels should be obtained on at least 2 separate days between 6 AM and 8 AM (preferably at the same time each day, eg., 8 AM). Plasma can be drawn and stored for ACTH measurements if deemed necessary. Stress or AM fasting cortisol levels that are less than 5 mg/dL are clearly abnormal and provide presumptive evidence of glucocorticoid deficiency (Figure 3). Stress or AM fasting cortisol levels of ≥5 mg/dL to <20 mg/dL are potentially abnormal. Stress or AM fasting cortisol values ≥20 mg/dL essentially exclude glucocorticoid insufficiency. In this later situation, it can be argued that further workup is not indicated. However if there is a clinical suspicion of glucocorticoid deficiency as in the above cases where the stress or AM cortisols are <20 mg/dL, a **One-Hour ACTH stimulation test** or an **ITT** should be performed. A peak cortisol of <20 mg/dL and a change in cortisol over baseline of <7 mg/dL (delta cortisol) are abnormal and are diagnostic for glucocorticoid deficiency. Further evaluation is indicated depending upon the clinical circumstances. For example, if the ACTH level is elevated at the time that the cortisol is low, primary adrenocortical insufficiency is highly likely and further testing may be unnecessary. If adrenal autoantibodies are detected associated with low stress or AM cortisol levels and an abnormal **One-hour ACTH Stimulation Test** or **ITT**, further testing should not be pursued because these results confirm autoimmune Addison disease.

Once a patient has been confirmed as having glucocorticoid deficiency, the **Two-Day ACTH Stimulation Test** is useful for differentiating primary glucocorticoid deficiency (primary adrenocortical failure, Addison disease) from secondary glucocorticoid deficiency (ACTH deficiency). When the adrenal gland is exposed to sustained exogenous ACTH stimulation, in cases of endogenous ACTH deficiency the adrenal gland will begin to produce cortisol. However in primary adrenocortical insufficiency, even with supraphysiologic exogenous ACTH stimulation the adrenal gland is unable to increase cortisol production. Thus an abnormal **Two-Day ACTH Stimulation Test** confirms *primary* glucocorticoid deficiency as there is a deficient cortisol response to ACTH even when maximal doses of ACTH are applied. In cases of Addison disease or ACTH deficiency, further confirmation that the hypothalamic-pituitary-adrenal axis is faulty can be achieved by performing **metyrapone testing.** The 3-4 day metyrapone test is the most widely used of the metyrapone tests presented (see tests of pituitary function chapter 1). Some investigators believe that metyrapone testing is the most sensitive approach to determining adrenal insufficiency. Patients might have normal basal values of cortisol and ACTH, normal responses to acute injections of exogenous ACTH, normal responses to insulin-induced hypoglycemia, and *yet* have deficient responses to metyrapone. If metyrapone testing is normal, it is unlikely that further testing is indicated.

Measuring ACTH levels may also assist in differentiating primary from secondary glucocorticoid deficiency. With primary glucocorticoid deficiency, ACTH would be elevated whereas in secondary glucocorticoid deficiency ACTH would be normal or depressed. However ACTH levels do not carry the same diagnostic weight as TSH levels in the evaluation of thyroid disease. ACTH is highly labile and its concentration is highly variable over the course of a day because of the normal diurnal variation that is observed in the hypothalamic-pituitary-adrenal axis.

ACTH deficiency is diagnosed when the **Two-day ACTH Stimulation Test** is normal yet the **One-hour ACTH Stimulation Test** or **ITT** are abnormal. ACTH deficiency can be primary (due to pituitary disease) or secondary (due to hypothalamic disease). As noted above, a normal or low concentration of ACTH concurrent with a depressed cortisol level in the morning or at a time of stress also supports the diagnosis of ACTH deficiency. Because the differentiation between hypothalamic and pituitary disease is usually accomplished radiographically, the CRH test is only rarely performed to differentiate primary from secondary ACTH deficiency.

If primary glucocorticoid deficiency (primary adrenocortical failure) is confirmed, evaluation of mineralocorticoid status is clearly indicated. Minimal evaluations include serum electrolytes and plasma renin activity (PRA) to define if there is: 1) normal mineralocorticoid function (normal electrolytes, normal PRA), 2) compensated mineralocorticoid deficiency (normal electrolytes, elevated PRA), or 3) uncompensated mineralocorticoid deficiency (hyponatremia, hypokalemia and elevated PRA).

3) Adrenal Function Tests

i) ACTH Stimulation Tests

The **One-Hour ACTH** (cortrosyn) **Stimulation Test** determines whether or not the adrenal cortex can respond to a single, acute pharmacologic dose of ACTH with an increase in cortisol production. If there is primary gland failure or gland atrophy from ACTH deficiency, peak cortisol following ACTH is <20 mg/dL and the change over baseline is <7 mg/dL. The absolute cortisol level is believed to be a better measure of glucocorticoid secretion than the change in cortisol over baseline. The 1 mg ACTH (cortrosyn) stimulation test must be considered experimental and is not recommended for routine use. The prolonged ACTH stimulation tests (**8-hour, Two-day and 3-5 Day ACTH Stimulation Tests**) provide higher levels of sustained ACTH stimulation to overcome adrenocortical atrophy that may have arisen from ACTH deficiency. With prolonged ACTH stimulation with primary adrenal failure, peak cortisol concentrations remain <20 mg/dL regardless of the extent or duration of ACTH administration. With ACTH or CRH deficiency, prolonged and sustained exogenous ACTH will stimulate the atrophied gland to redevelop and produce a cortisol response of ≥20mg/dL.

ii) The One-Hour ACTH Stimulation Test

ACTH (cosyntropin or cortrosyn) is administered intravenously or intramuscularly (25 units or 250 mg) as a bolus(1). Cosyntropin is a 1-24 corticotropin that is sold as Cortrosyn^{R} (Organon, Inc., Liberty Corner, NJ). Prior to injection, a baseline cortisol is measured along with samples taken at +30 and +60 minutes. Outside the U.S., ACTH(1-18) amide is sometimes used. If only one post-ACTH sample is obtained, it can be drawn at +45 minutes. If the adrenal cortex has normal function, the stimulated cortisol is ≥20 mg/dL and the change over baseline is ≥7 (to ≥10) mg/dL. Between the two criteria, the absolute cortisol level is more important. If the basal cortisol is ≥20 mg/dL, ACTH administration may produce little further elevation in serum cortisol because the patient may already be maximally stimulated at baseline.

Be aware that with acute ACTH or CRH deficiency, the serum cortisol response to stress is low while the adrenal cortex's response to exogenous ACTH is normal. Several weeks or months must pass after ACTH or CRH deficiency initially develops before the adrenal cortex atrophies. *If there is an abnormal serum cortisol in response to stress and a normal ACTH stimulation test when acute ACTH or CRH deficiency is a clinical possibility, an insulin tolerance test or metyrapone test should be performed.*

iii) 8-Hour, Two-Day And 3-5 Day ACTH Stimulation Tests

When ACTH or CRH deficiency are suspected and the physician wants to prove that the adrenal gland has otherwise normal function, a *prolonged ACTH stimulation test* is performed. There are several variations that strive to provide sufficient ACTH to reverse any atrophy that has developed from ACTH or CRH inadequacy.

In the 8 hour test, a baseline 24 urine sample for urinary free cortisol (UFC) is measured. Assessment of UFC provides an integrated 24 hour measurement of cortisol production. On day two, a 24-hour urine collection is begun and Cortrosyn is delivered intravenously (25 units or 250 mg) with the infusion completed in eight hours. The cortisol at +60 minutes should be >20 mg/dL and at +8 hours, ≥25 mg/dL. UFC on day two should be ≥3 fold greater compared to the baseline collection.

The Two-Day and 3-5 day tests deliver Cortrosyn every day (an infusion over 8 hours or via IM injection, or a continuous infusion of ACTH) with similar expected increases in cortisol and UFC. Presently, the two-day test is the most popular prolonged ACTH stimulation test (one day of baseline urine collection and two days of continuous ACTH administration).

With endogenous ACTH or CRH deficiency, the 8-hour test may not be long enough to elicit a normal cortisol response. After maximal exogenous ACTH stimulation, if cortisol does not increase appropriately (eg., ≥20 mg/dL), primary adrenal insufficiency is confirmed. Finding an elevated basal ACTH is consistent with a primary failure of cortisol production.

iv) Mineralocorticoid Assessment

Aldosterone concentrations vary with salt intake and body position. Salt restriction can raise aldosterone levels ≥8 fold. To account for such wide variations, it is good practice to collect a 24-hour urine for sodium excretion. Aldosterone reference ranges can then be related to salt intake. Urine creatinine is measured to monitor completeness of collection and should be measured on all timed urine collections.

Prior to the measurement of basal serum aldosterone concentrations, patients should be supine for 30 minutes and on their normal salt intake for 24 to 48 hours. Standing can double aldosterone concentrations. Alternatively, a 24 hour urine can be collected for aldosterone excretion to assess an integrated measurement of aldosterone production. With deficient secretion of aldosterone, normally there is an increase in PRA (plasma renin activity).

On a normal sodium intake, aldosterone excretion is 3-10 mg/day. Values of 20-50 mg/day are achieved with a low salt diet. If the diagnosis of mineralocorticoid deficiency is in question, plasma aldosterone and PRA should be obtained after 3 hours of upright posture or after a day or more of salt restriction (e.g, a low salt diet). Normally with such measures, aldosterone and PRA rise. Salt restriction should be undertaken with care so as not to precipitate Addisonian crisis.

If frank electrolyte disturbances are lacking, it is reasonable to perform these tests of mineralocorticoid function in patients under evaluation for primary adrenocortical failure. On the other hand, if the patient has a history suggestive of mineralocorticoid deficiency and manifests hyponatremia, hyperkalemia, and a normal anion gap metabolic acidosis, aldosterone need not be measured. If required for diagnosis, low serum aldosterone, low urinary excretion of aldosterone, and elevated PRA are strong evidence of primary adrenal insufficiency.

Aldosterone deficiency is treated with florinef (9α-fluorohydrocortisone). Patients with mineralocorticoid deficiency who are undertreated can display electrolyte abnormalities as described above and hypertension from elevated PRA and angiotensin II that causes vasoconstrition. In contrast with severe untreated mineralocorticoid deficiency, hypotension can quickly supervene followed by shock or death.

D) Congenital Adrenal Hyperplasia

The most common cause of adrenocortical insufficiency in the newborn period is congenital adrenal hyperplasia (CAH). Rarely, adrenal failure occurs from traumatic adrenal hemorrhage or adrenal hemorrhage from sepsis. CAH results from various inborn errors in the biosynthesis of cortisol. With deficient cortisol production, ACTH levels rise and anatomically cause the adrenal hyperplasia for which CAH is named. The two most common causes of CAH are 21-hydroxylase deficiency (CYP21 deficiency) and 11ß-hydroxylase deficiency (CYP11B1 deficiency) (see Figure 2 for biosynthetic pathway).

21-Hydroxylase is normally responsible for the conversion of progesterone to desoxycorticosterone (DOC) in the zona glomerulosa and 17-hydroxyprogesterone (17-OHP) to desoxycortisol in the zona fasiculata. 11ß-hydroxylase normally catalyzes the conversion of desoxycorticosterone to corticosterone in the zona glomerulosa and desoxycortisol to cortisol in the zona fasiculata. Either defect results in deficient cortisol production, eliciting a rise in ACTH concentrations. In turn, because of ACTH excess and the metabolic blocks in cortisol biosynthesis, the adrenal androgens dehydroepiandrosterone (DHEA) and androstenedione are overproduced. In females overproduction of the adrenal androgens induces virilization in utero. In males, adrenal androgen overproduction produces precocious puberty. Untreated, postnatal females will continue to virilize. The more profound the defect in cortisol biosynthesis, the greater the elevation in ACTH and greater the degree of virilization in the female fetus or precocious puberty in males and virilization in post-natal females. Virilization in females can vary from mild fusion of the labia, to marked labial fusion with clitoromegaly, to complete masculinization with male external genitalia, with the exception of bilaterally undescended "testes," which in reality are ovaries that are in their normal intra-abdominal location.

Glucocorticoid insufficiency leads to malaise, failure to thrive, hypoglycemia, and vascular instability. In approximately one half of infants affected with 21-hydroxylase deficiency CAH, in addition to deficient cortisol production, there is deficient mineralocorticoid production that can cause hyponatremia, hyperkalemia, acidosis, dehydration, and hypotension. In its most severe form, this type of "salt-losing" 21-hydroxylase deficiency CAH clinically presents at 10 to 14 days of age with Addisonian crisis. Because salt-losing 21-hydroxylase CAH is a more severe expression of the inborn error than non-salt-losing 21-hydroxylase deficiency CAH, salt-losing 21-hydroxylase deficiency CAH is associated with more severe degrees of virilization in males and females. Untreated, mortality is very high in salt-losing 21-hydroxylase deficiency CAH.

In summary in 21-hydroxylase deficiency CAH, females can present with ambiguous genitalia, post-natal virilization, or neonatal salt-losing Addisonian crisis. Males present with precocious puberty during infancy or childhood or neonatal salt losing crisis.

In the case of 11ß-hydroxylase deficiency CAH, there is overproduction of DOC because of the block in the conversion of DOC to corticosterone. DOC has mineralocorticoid activity. Whereas girls with 11ß-hydroxylase deficiency present with ambiguous genitalia and boys display precocious puberty, salt loss does not occur in 11ß-hydroxylase deficiency. Therefore, electrolyte disturbances and acidosis do not occur nor does Addisonian crisis develop in the newborn period. In later childhood, elevated DOC can produce hypermineralocorticoidism and hypokalemic hypertension, which is discussed in more detail below.

The diagnosis of 21-hydroxylase deficiency and 11ß-hydroxylase deficiency is dependent upon finding elevated concentrations of 17-OHP in plasma or serum. In addition, 21-hydroxylase deficiency and 11ß-hydroxylase deficiency can be differentiated using measurements of urinary 17-hydroxycorticosteroids or desoxycortisol. Elevated pregnanetriol excretion in the urine reflects elevated 17-OHP concentrations in the blood stream (Figure 4). Both disorders display elevated urinary 17-ketogenic steroids (17-KGS). The 17-KGS are urinary breakdown products of 17-hydroxyprogesterone, desoxycortisol, and cortisol. The urinary 17-hydroxycorticosteroids (17-OHCS) are breakdown products desoxycortisol and cortisol. In 11ß-hydroxylase deficiency, 17-OHCS are elevated, whereas in 21-hydroxylase deficiency 17-OHCS are not elevated because the 21-hydroxylase metabolic block inhibits production of both desoxycortisol and cortisol. In 21-hydroxylase deficiency, both desoxycortisol and cortisol are low, while in 11ß-hydroxylase deficiency, desoxycortisol is elevated and cortisol is low. The urinary 17-ketosteroids (17-KS) are breakdown products of the adrenal androgens dehydroepiandrosterone (DHEA) and androstenedione. Testosterone does not contribute to the formation of 17-KS. In both disorders, DHEA, androstenedione, and 17-KS are elevated. These results are compared in Table 1.

A "late-onset" or "attenuated" (nonclassical) form of 21-hydroxylase deficiency [that is much milder than the classical ("virilizing") form of 21-hydroxylase deficiency of prenatal onset] can present in female adolescents as hirsutism or virilization. Whereas baseline and post-ACTH (see cortrosyn stimulation test) 17-OHP levels in attenutated 21-hydroxylase deficient CAH are higher than in controls, the values are not as high as those seen in classical 21-hydroxylase deficiency CAH. Graphs are available in the literature that allow basal 17-OHP to be plotted against post-ACTH 17-OHP in diagnosing CAH gene carriers versus attentuated 21-hydroxylase deficiency versus classical 21-hydroxylase deficiency.

CAH patients may be followed clinically by measuring an early AM

FIGURE 4. URINARY STEROIDS ASSAYED IN THE DIAGNOSIS AND MANAGEMENT OF CAH

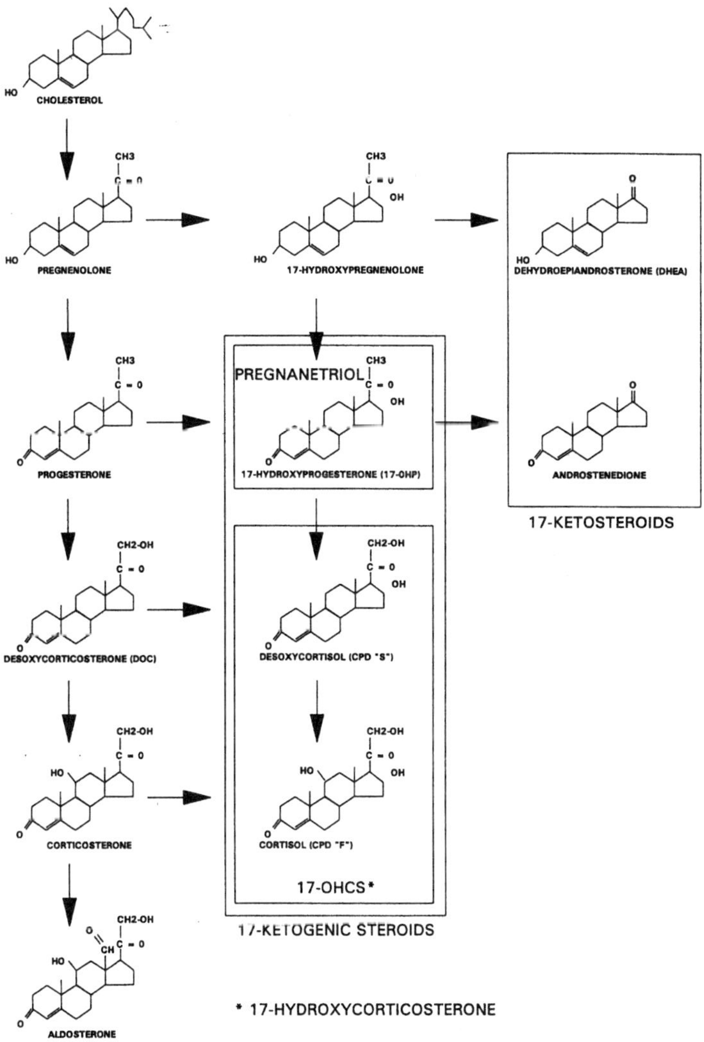

The 17-ketogenic steroids (17-KGS) are urinary breakdown products of 17-hydroxyprogesterone, desoxycortisol, and cortisol. The urinary 17-hydroxycorticosteroids (17-OHCS) are breakdown products desoxycortisol and cortisol. The urinary 17-ketosteroids (17-KS) are breakdown products of the adrenal androgens dehydroepiandrosterone (DHEA) and androstenedione. Testosterone does not contribute to the formation of 17-KS.

Table 1: Comparison of 21-hydroxylase deficient and 11ß-hydroxylase deficient forms of CAH

	ENZYME DEFICIENCY 21-HYDROXYLASE	11ß-HYDROXYLASE
Gene	CYP21	CYP11B1
17-OHP	Elevated	Elevated
DOC	Depressed	Elevated
Corticosterone	Depressed	Depressed
Desoxycortisol	Depressed	Elevated
Cortisol	Depressed*	Depressed*
17-KGS	Elevated	Elevated
17-OHCS	Depressed	Elevated
17-KS	Elevated	Elevated
Ambiguous genitalia	In females	In females
Precocious puberty	In boys	In boys
Salt loss	Present in ~1/2 of patients	No
Hypertension	No	Late childhood/adolescence

* *In mild forms of CAH, cortisol may be low normal from a compensatory elevation in ACTH*

17-OHP or androstenedione at any time of the day. The treatment is cortisol replacement. Aldosterone is replaced as described above with fluorinef. With adequate glucocorticoid replacement, 17-OHP or androstenedione should not be elevated above the upper limit of normal. Under-replacement with glucocorticoids can allow excess adrenal androgen production and post-natal virilization, accelerated growth, premature closure of the epiphyses, and short stature. Over-treatment with glucocorticoids can produce poor growth from iatrogenic Cushing syndrome.

II) Adrenocortical Excess

A) Clinical Symptoms of Glucocorticoid Excess

The symptoms of Cushing syndrome [glucocorticoid (cortisol) excess] include weight gain, weakness, menstrual irregularities/impotence, back pain, psychological changes, and headache. The signs include "moon-shaped" facies, acne, thoracic kyphosis, supraclavicular fat pad, hypertrichosis, purplish stria, psychosis, easy bruising, hypertension, buffalo hump, and centripetal obesity. Excess cortisol may produce glucose intolerance or frank diabetes. Severe myopathy (muscle disorder) can be noted as proximal muscle weakness. With concomitant oversecretion of adrenal androgens, women can experience hirsutism or virilization. Non-endocrine laboratory findings can encompass alkalosis, hypokalemia, elevated hematocrit, and eosinopenia.

With chronic elevations in ACTH concentration, hyperpigmentation results because of MSH-like (melanocyte stimulating hormone-like) activity of ACTH. Marked cortisol excess can also lead to salt and water retention with electrolyte problems similar to aldosterone excess. Because of its potent antiinflammatory effects, blunting of the immune response predisposes to infection. Ostcopenia in adults and poor linear growth in children result from excess cortisol. Peptic ulcer can also develop.

Excessive mineralocorticoid action from hyperaldosteronism or excessive cortisol secretion produces hypokalemia, systemic alkalosis (hypochloremia and high HCO_3^- concentration), and hypertension from sodium and water retention with expansion of circulating blood volume. Conn's syndrome is the clinical expression of an aldosterone (mineralocorticoid)-secreting adrenal tumor (e.g., an aldosteronoma).

B) The Differential Diagnosis of Glucocorticoid Excess

Cushing syndrome results from: 1) ACTH-independent hypercortisolism from autonomous overproduction of cortisol by the adrenal gland (eg., adrenocortical adenoma or carcinoma; micronodular dysplasia, or macronodular hyperplasia) or excessive exogenous administration of glucocorticoids (iatrogenic or factitious Cushing syndrome), or by 2) inappropriate or excessive secretion of ACTH (ACTH-dependent hypercortisolism). Macronodular hyperplasia is very rare.

Excessive ACTH secretion (ACTH-dependent hypercortisolism) can result from a pituitary tumor (Cushing disease), or from a non-pituitary tumor overproducing ACTH (ectopic ACTH syndrome) or CRH (ectopic CRH syndrome).

C) The Biochemical Diagnosis of Glucocorticoid Excess

To establish the laboratory diagnosis of Cushing syndrome, excess cortisol secretion must be confirmed. The approach outlined below is believed to be reasonable and expeditious (Figure 5). For Cushing syndrome there is no one test strategy that is agreed upon by all endocrinologists. Before beginning such a biochemical evaluation, it is important for the clinical team to outline their plan of diagnostic "attack."

1) Serum Cortisol and ACTH Measurements

Diurnal variation is lost when the PM cortisol level is inappropriately

FIGURE 5. CLINICALLY SUSPECTED CUSHING SYNDROME

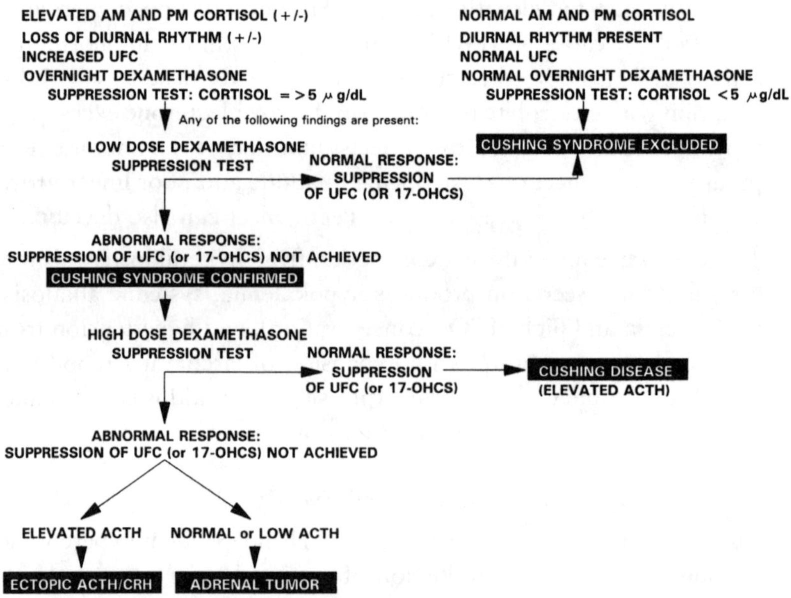

When Cushing syndrome is suspected and supported by urinary free cortisol (UFC) or other measurements, a low-dose dexamethasone suppression test should be performed. If abnormal or as a continuation of the initial test, a high-dose dexamethasone suppression test is classically performed. Failure to suppress on high-dose dexamethasone is consistent with adrenal tumor or ectopic ACTH that are evaluated by CT or MRI of the adrenal glands and measurement of ACTH.

elevated (eg., PM value ≥~50% of the AM level). Several abnormal patterns of plasma cortisol secretion may be observed in Cushing syndrome: 1) Elevated AM and PM cortisol (with or without loss of diurnal variation), or 2) Normal AM, but elevated PM concentrations (loss of diurnal variation). In Cushing syndrome, random cortisol levels are rarely <7 mg/dL. The usual range for cortisol in Cushing syndrome is 15-35 mg/dL regardless of the time of the day.

If serum cortisol is to be measured in the evaluation of patients with suspected Cushing syndrome, the PM levels are much more informative than the AM levels in search of loss of diurnal variation. However, only about 60% of patients with Cushing syndrome display a loss of diurnal variation. PM cortisol levels should be obtained at ~1 AM (or one hour after retiring to bed) on at least two days. If drawn, AM cortisols should be obtained between 6 AM and 8 AM. One AM cortisol levels are normally usually <5 mg/dL. Typical reference ranges for AM cortisol levels are 7 to 25 mg/dL and for PM values (8 to 10 PM), 2 to 9 mg/dL.

Some authors advise against measuring serum cortisol levels (even PM levels) and recommend proceeding directly to measurement of urinary free cortisol (UFC) when the diagnosis of Cushing syndrome is under consideration. On the other hand, a faulty 24-hour urine collection is not useful and in such a situation serum cortisol levels would be the next most valuable tools. UFC can be corrected for body surface area or body weight in an attempt to correct for exogenous obesity or large body size. UFC measured by non-HPLC methods is unreliable because of cross-reactivity with other steroids.

The finding of an elevated UFC in a 24-hour urine specimen documents overproduction of cortisol. Two baseline 24-hour samples should be obtained to take into consideration day-to-day variation in steroid secretion. UFC values of ≥70 $mg/m^2/day$ suggest Cushing syndrome, assuming that the samples are not obtained during periods of high stress (e.g., trauma or surgery).

As ACTH measurements are helpful in the differential diagnosis of Cushing syndrome, ACTH could be measured at 1 AM on two separate nights at the same time the PM cortisol values are drawn. Normally, ACTH at this time should be <10 pg/mL. To avoid any effects of stress-induced phlebotomy on steroid hormone or ACTH secretion, an indwelling catheter should be introduced hours prior to any sampling that is performed and kept open with a dilute heparin solution or heparin lock.

2) Overnight Dexamethasone Suppression Test

After evaluation of serum cortisol and UFC, if the biochemical diagnosis of Cushing syndrome is still unclear, an **overnight dexamethasone suppression test** should be carried out. In this investigation, 1 mg of dexamethasone is given orally at 10 PM. At 8 AM the following morning, a fasting cortisol is measured. A normal response is indicated by a serum cortisol concentration of <5 mg/dL demonstrating that the hypothalamic-pituitary-adrenal axis can be suppressed with administration of exogenous glucocorticoid. Dexamethasone is used because it does not cross-react in the typical cortisol immunoassay. Equivocal responses are noted as cortisol levels of 5 to 9.9 mg/dL. 8 AM cortisols of ≥10 mg/dL are abnormal and are consistent with Cushing syndrome. The overnight dexamethasone suppression test has a high sensitivity for detecting Cushing syndrome (~>95%). However the test is not highly specific, as there is a 10 to 15% false-positive rate (failure of suppression in the absence of Cushing syndrome). False positives can result from failure to take dexamethasone, or increased dexamethasone metabolism, and episodic ACTH secretion. False negatives are unusual and could result from delayed metabolism of dexamethasone.

D) Diagnostic Workup For Glucocorticoid Excess

1) Low-Dose Dexamethasone Suppression Test

For patients that have clear elevations in the excretion of urinary glucocorticoids (e.g., elevated UFC ± collaborated by elevated serum cortisol levels), or in patients with 8 AM cortisols ≥5 mg/dL after overnight dexamethasone suppression, a **low-dose dexamethasone suppression** test is next performed. In this test, two baseline 24 hour urines are collected for 17-hydroxycorticosteroids (17-OHCS) or UFC (days 1 and 2). On days 3 and 4, 0.5 mg (1.25 mg/m^2) of dexamethasone is given orally every 6 hours for a total of 8 doses. With Cushing syndrome, there is no significant suppression of 17-OHCS or UFC on low-dose dexamethasone: the 17-OHCS or UFC on days 3 or 4 of low-dose dexamethasone do not decline to <50% of the mean baseline (day 1 and 2) values (mg excreted per 24 hrs).

In normal individuals, six hours after the last dose of dexamethasone, serum cortisol should be <5 mg/dL and ACTH should be <20 pg/mL, whereas 17-OHCS are <4 mg per 24 hrs and UFC is <25 mg per 24 hrs. Cushing syndrome is confirmed when UFC on days 3 or 4 are more than 50% of the baseline value. An absolute UFC of ≥25 mg/day while on low dose dexamethasone also supports the diagnosis of Cushing syndrome. Therefore in summary a baseline absolute elevation in UFC excretion is consistent with glucocorticoid excess (Cushing syndrome) and is confirmed by failure of UFC suppression on low dose dexamethasone.

2) High-Dose Dexamethasone Suppression Test

When the low-dose dexamethasone suppression test is abnormal [e.g., Cushing syndrome (glucocorticoid excess) is confirmed], a **high-dose dexamethasone suppression test** is performed. This test is similar to the low-dose test except that 2 mg (3.75 mg/m^2) of dexamethasone are administered every 6 hours instead of 0.5 mg. In normal individuals, similar to low-dexamethasone suppression, with high-dose dexamethasone suppresion 17-OHCS and UFC should decline by >50% of baseline values.

The high-dose test may be helpful in differentiating Cushing disease *from* adrenal tumor or ectopic ACTH/CRH syndrome. However, this test does not correctly classify all patients. Cushing disease is a subtype of Cushing syndrome that results from a pituitary corticotroph microadenoma. When the patient is treated with high-dose dexamethasone, in Cushing disease the 17-OHCS or UFC are usually (but not always) suppressed to values <50% of baseline values. On the other hand, adrenal tumor and ectopic ACTH demonstrate a decline in 17-OHCS or UFC of <50%. As with the low-dose dexamethasone suppression test, some endocrinologists may order urinary 17-hydroxycorticosteroids (17-OHCS) in place of UFC, but it can be argued that UFC is a more "specific" measure of cortisol production than 17-OHCS.

In cases of Cushing disease, the pituitary microadenoma has a raised plasma cortisol set point for negative feedback. Some cases of Cushing syndrome require still higher doses of dexamethasone to demonstrate suppression (e.g., 16 mg or more per day). The high-dose dexamethasone suppression test can be run on days 5 and 6 immediately following the low-dose dexamethasone suppression test, eliminating the need for repeated baseline laboratory studies of UFC, cortisol, and ACTH.

3) ACTH Measurements

When high-dose dexamethasone fails to suppress UFC excretion, adrenal tumor and ectopic ACTH/CRH syndrome must be differentiated. If ACTH measurements were obtained during the patient's initial evaluation, ACTH should be suppressed by autonomous cortisol production by an adrenal tumor. In contrast, ACTH is measurable or elevated in Cushing disease or ectopic ACTH/CRH syndrome. Assuming that the ACTH is below the reference range and there is failure of UFC suppression with high dose dexamethasone, radiographic imaging studies for an adrenal tumor should be pursued (e.g., MRI or CAT scan, etc.).

Assuming that the ACTH is measurable or elevated with failure of UFC suppression with high dose dexamethasone, ectopic ACTH/CRH syndrome is sought by investigating the patient for an underlying tumor (e.g., oat cell carcinoma of the lung or carcinoid). The expected results for plasma ACTH, low-dose and high-dose dexamethasone suppression tests are summarized in Table 2.

TABLE 2: TYPICAL LABORATORY FINDINGS IN CUSHING SYNDROME

ETIOLOGY	ACTH LOW DOSE	DEXAMETHASONE SUPPRESSION TEST*	HIGH DOSE DEXAMETHASONE SUPPRESSION TEST*
Cushing disease	↑	No suppression	Suppression achieved
Ectopic ACTH/ CRH Syndrome	↑	No suppression	No suppression
Adrenal tumor	↓	No suppression	No suppression

↑ *Increased;* ↓ *Decreased; *17-OHCS or UFC*

4) Inferior Petrosal Sinus Sampling (IPSS) for ACTH Following CRH

Biochemical evidence of Cushing disease (an ACTH-producing pituitary tumor) indicates the need for radiographic pituitary evaluation (e.g., CT or MRI). If the source of ACTH is equivocal, e.g., pituitary versus extrapituitary when a pituitary tumor cannot be definitively visualized radiographically, a CRH stimulation test can be performed with simultaneous bilateral petrosal venous sampling (4-6). With a pituitary microadenoma, CRH will elicit an increase in ACTH while in ectopic ACTH, pituitary ACTH will be suppressed. Comparison with a simultaneous peripheral ACTH measurement confirms (or denies) ACTH release from the pituitary. Samples at all three sites are obtained at baseline (-15 minutes and 0 minutes) and at +15 and +30 minutes following bolus administration of intravenous CRH (eg., 100 mg/m^2). The average IPSS ACTH to peripheral ACTH gradient in Cushing disease is 15 with the lower limit of normal near 1.5 to 1.7 Contrary to early reports, IPSS sampling for ACTH following CRH is a poor predictor of the side of the pituitary gland that harbors the ACTH-producing microadenoma.

E) Hypermineralocorticoidism

Adrenal tumors may overproduce mineralocorticoids (e.g., aldosteronomas) and not glucocorticoids. As noted previously, Conn syndrome results from an adrenal tumor solely overproducing aldosterone that causes hypertension from salt and water retention. In Conn syndrome glucocorticoid excess and clinical stigmata of Cushing syndrome are absent. Alkalosis and hypokalemia accompanied by hypertension in cases of mineralocorticoid excess should be evaluated by measuring serum and/or urine aldosterone and plasma renin activity (PRA). With autonomous overproduction of mineralocorticoid, serum and urine aldosterone are elevated while PRA is suppressed.

In the renin assay, the ability of plasma to generate angiotensin I from angiotensinogen present in the patient's own plasma constitutes the "plasma renin activity (PRA)." Angiotensin I is measured by immunoradiometric assay (IRMA). Contrary to the policy in many laboratories, plasma should *not* be cooled prior to being spun, separated, and frozen. Placing plasma on ice can actually falsely raise PRA as cold will "cryoactivate" prorenin to renin. The concentration of prorenin can exceed that of renin by a factor of 10. Renin can also be measured by immunoassay. However, PRA is considered by many to be a superior assay because the incubation time for angiotensin I generation can be extended to measure low PRAs. Usually PRA and renin measured by IRMA are highly correlated.

Measurement of urinary sodium excretion can help profile the patient's PRA measurement (Table 3). Figure 1 summarized the physiology of the renin-angiotensin-aldosterone system. Depressed PRA is observed with primary hyperaldosteronism, hyporeninemic hypoaldosteronism (as seen in association with diabetes mellitus), following bilateral nephrectomy, in low renin essential hypertension, with licorice or mineralocorticoid ingestion, and with administration of certain drugs (e.g., ß blockers, clonidine, and DOC).

When hypokalemia is first identified in any hypertensive patient, hypokalemia due to diuretics (e.g., thiazides or furosemide) must be excluded before a complex evaluation for excessive mineralocorticoid action is pursued (Figure 6). Potassium-wasting diuretics should be discontinued for 2 months before serum potassium is measured for diagnostic

Table 3: Sample Reference Ranges for Peripheral Renin Activity (PRA; ng/mL/hr; assay performed at pH 6)

PATIENT CONDITION	REFERENCE RANGE	COMMENT
Random	0.84 - 2.50	This value is difficult to apply; supine PRAs are more interpretable
Nonambulatory	1.45 - 5.15	PRA is frequently higher in chronically ill pateints and hospitalized patients because of intercurrent disease
Supine	0.15 - 2.33	Patient should be supine for ≥30 minutes
Erect	0.131 - 3.95	Supine values are more informative for the diagnosis of hyperreninism
Urinary Sodium Excretion*		Sodium intake has a marked effect on the PRA
0-30	8.8-23.9	Sodium restriction normally increases the PRA
30-75	4.1-7.7	Sodium restriction normally increases the PRA
75-150	1.44-2.8	Note: PRAs in infants and children are higher than
>150	0.39-1.31	in adults (use age adjusted reference ranges)

**mEq per 24 hours*

purposes. Patients on angiotensin-converting enzyme (ACE) blockers may have a falsely normal potassium and such drugs must also be discontinued prior to "potassium" profiling.

In the distal convoluted tubule, hypermineralocorticoidism causes sodium (and water) retention in exchange for hydrogen ion and potassium wasting into the urine. These later events produce a metabolic alkalosis and hypokalemia. Urinary potassium is typically elevated at >30 meq/L. In the absence of hypermineralocorticoidism, the kidney will conserve potassium in the face of systemic hypokalemia. While the major stimulator of aldosterone secretion is angiotensin II, aldosterone is also stimulated to lesser degrees by hypokalemia and ACTH.

Volume expansion from hypermineralocorticoidism produces elevations in blood pressure. Vasoconstriction from elevated angiotensin II levels also occurs when renin is elevated. Excessive mineralocorticoid action results from 1) high renin concentrations activating the angiotensin-al-

FIGURE 6. HYPERTENSION WITH A LOW SERUM POTASSIUM

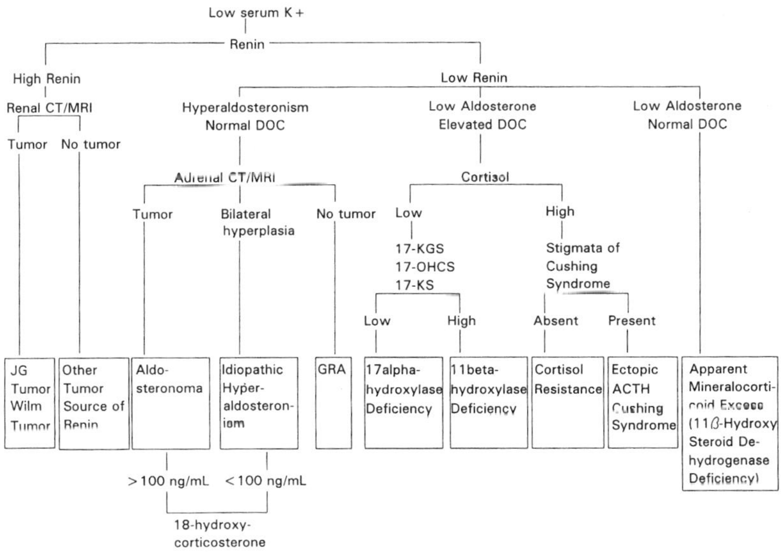

Hypertension and hypokalemia (in the absence of potassium-wasting diuretic use) identifies patients with hypermineralocorticoidism. Renin measurement separates this group into hyperreninemic hyperaldosteronism versus hyporeninemic hypermineralocorticoidism. With hyperreninemic hyperaldosteronism, the source of the renin secretion must be identified. Note that with severe renovascular hypertension, hyperreninemic hyperaldosteronism and hypokalemia can result (this is not noted in figure 6). With hyporeninemic hypermineralocorticoidism, the hypermineralocorticoidism can result from 1) elevated aldosterone secretion [e.g., primary hyperaldosteronism] with normal desoxycorticosterone (DOC), 2) elevated DOC secretion from elevated ACTH levels [e.g., congenital adrenal hyperplasia (CAH), cortisol resistance, or ectopic ACTH secretion] with suppressed aldosterone, or 3) local excessive mineralocorticoid effect from 11β-hydroxysteroid dehydrogenase deficiency in mineralocorticoid-sensitive tissues (e.g., the distal convoluted tubule). Primary hyperaldosteronism can result from an adrenal aldosterone-secreting tumor (an aldosteronoma), bilateral adrenal hyperplasia (idiopathic hyperaldosteronism), or glucocorticoid-remediable aldosteronism (also known as dexamethasone-supppressible hypertension). CT or MRI can help differentiate these later 3 conditions. Measurement of 18-hydroxycorticosterone can also assist in differentiating an aldosteronoma from bilateral hyperplasia. Two forms of CAH can produce hypertension: 17α-hydroxylase deficiency and 11β-hydroxylase deficiency. Patients with cortisol resistance have biochemical hypercortisolism but few if any clinical features of Cushing syndrome.

dosterone axis (primary hyperreninism), 2) primary mineralocorticoid excess [primary hyperaldosteronism (aldosteronoma, idiopathic primary hyperaldosteronism, glucocorticoid remediable aldosteronism), or elevated deoxycorticosterone concentrations (17α-hydroxylase deficiency, 11ß-hydroxylase deficiency, cortisol resistance, ectopic ACTH causing Cushing syndrome)], or 3) local excessive mineralocorticoid action (apparent mineralocorticoid excess) (Table 4). Aldosterone biosynthesis from progesterone is outlined below.

progesterone
•
• 21-hydroxylase activity of CYP21
▽
desoxycorticosterone (DOC)
•
• 11ß-hydroxylase activity of CYP11B1
▽
corticosterone
•
• 18-hydroxylase activity of CYP11B2
▽
18-hydroxycorticosterone
•
• 18-oxidase activity of CYP11B2
▽
aldosterone

1) Hyperreninic Hyperaldosteronism

If hypokalemia and hyperreninism are identified, a source for the elevated renin production must be identified. Renovascular disease should be investigated (e.g., a captopril stimulation test). If a renal CT or MRI reveals a mass, a juxtaglomerular tumor (renal hemangiopericytoma), Wilm tumor, or other renal tumor (e.g., renal adenocarcinoma) must be excluded. Otherwise, extra-renal tumors as sources of renin must be sought, e.g., an ovarian cancer in women, pancreatic adenocarcinoma, adenocarcinoma and small-cell tumor of the lung, adrenocortical carcinoma, and angiolymphoid hyperplasia with eosinophilia.

TABLE 4 : DIFFERENTIAL DIAGNOSIS OF HYPOKALEMIC HYPERTENSION (HTN): FUNCTIONAL HYPERALDOSTERONISM

CONDITION	K^+	RENIN	ALDO.	DOC	CT/ MRI: MASS	CORTISOL	OTHER COMMENTS/INVESTIGATIONS
Primary Hyperaldosteronism							
Aldosteronoma	↓	↓	↑	Nl	+		Renal vein sampling reveals unilateral increase in aldo., no increase in aldo. in response to upright posture; however if aldo. rises with upright posture, the diagnosis is "renin-responsive" aldosterenoma; Conn syndrome or APA: aldosterone-producing adrenal adenoma; 18-hydroxycorticosterone elevated
Idiopathic 1° hyperaldosteronism	↓	↓	↑	Nl	–		Increase in aldo. in response to upright posture; bilateral hyperplasia; 18-hydroxycorticosterone not elevated
Glucocorticoid remediable aldosteronism (GRA)	↓	↓	↑	Nl	–		Autosomal dominant, early-onset, HTN corrected by glucocorticoid replacement
Elevated DOC							
17α-hydroxylase deficiency	↓	↓	↓	↑	–	↓	Phenotypic female who fails to enter puberty or estrogenize; urinary 17-OHCS, 17-KGS, and 17-KS are low, cortisol is deficient
11ß-hydroxylase deficiency	↓	↓	↓	↑	–	↓	Adrenal androgen excess causes precocious puberty in boys and ambiguous genitalia in girls; urinary 17-OHCS, 17-KGS, and 17-KS are high
Cortisol resistance	↓	↓	↓	↑	–	↑	Cortisol is elevated (serum and urinary free cortisol) without clinical evidence of Cushing syndrome, ACTH is elevated
Ectopic ACTH Cushing	↓	↓	↓	↑	+	↑	Elevated $U_{cortisol}$, serum cortisol, etc., ACTH elevated
11ß-HSD deficiency (AME)	↓	↓	↓	Nl	–	Nl	Increased ratio of THF to THE
JG, Wilm tumor	↓	↑	↑	(Nl)	+	Nl	Renal mass, unilateral increased renin excretion
Extra-renal renin secreting	↓	↑	↑	(Nl)	+	Nl	Flank mass in a child suggests Wilm tumor; adnexal mass and tumor carcinomatosis in a women raises the possibility of ovarian cancer

Aldo. = aldosterone; AME = apparent mineralocorticoid excess; DOC = desoxyxorticosterone; HTN = hypertension

2) Primary Hyperaldosteronism

Besides observing absolute elevations in either serum or urinary aldosterone in hyperaldosteronism, calcuation of the aldosterone to renin ratio can be helpful in identifying hyperaldosteronism with concurrent renin suppression (situations of low serum potassium, high aldosterone, and low renin). Aldosterone (ng/dL) to renin (ng/mL/hr) ratios of >20-25 indicate hyperaldosteronism with relative suppression of renin (e.g., primary hyperaldosteronism). Primary hyperaldosteronism occurs in ~0.3% of adults with hypertension. Aldosteronomas may be visualized by CT or MRI. These tumors produce serum concentrations of 18-hydroxycorticosterone of >100 ng/dL which likely reflects inefficiency of aldosterone production by the tumor. On the other hand, 18-hydroxycorticosterone is <100 ng/dL in idiopathic primary hyperaldosteronism which may appear as bilateral hyperplasia on CT or MRI. With adrenal vein sampling by venography, a unilateral preponderance of 18-hydroxycorticosterone and an increase in 18-hydroxycorticosterone after cortrosyn help localize the aldosteronoma to a particular adrenal gland. In aldosteronoma, the aldosterone from the involved adrenal is very high while the contralateral adrenal aldosterone will be suppressed. In "idiopathic-bilateral hyperplasic" hyperaldosteronism, aldosterone in both adrenal veins is elevated and a high differential from one side to the other does not exist as is the case with aldosteronoma. Only 1-2% of aldosteronomas are malignant.

Another differential tool is that aldosterone concentrations do not usually rise with upright posture in aldosteronoma whereas aldosterone does rise with upright posture in idiopathic primary hyperaldosteronism. However measuring aldosterone changes with changes in posture is not infallible: there are unusual renin-responsive aldosteronomas where aldosterone increases with upright posture. Renin-responsive aldosteronomas emphasize the need for careful radiologic imaging studies.

3) Glucocorticoid-Remediable Aldosteronism

In primary hyperaldosteronism (elevated aldosterone production and suppressed PRA) when tumor and bilateral hyperplasia have been excluded, glucocorticoid-remediable aldosteronism (GRA) should be considered. This is an autosomal dominant disorder characterized by youth-onset hypertension and stroke. GRA is caused by ectopic expression of CYP11B2 activity (aldosterone synthase activity) in the fasiculata with mineralocorticoid production falling under control of ACTH, leading to mineralocorticoid overproduction. Normally, CYP11B1 is the gene that encodes the

11ß-hydroxylase that is expressed in the adrenal zona fasiculata that is under ACTH control (e.g., the CYP11B1 promoter is stimulated by ACTH). 11ß-Hydroxylase is responsible for the conversion of desoxycortisol to cortisol. Expressed in the adrenal zona glomerulosa, CYP11B2 is the gene that encodes 18-hydroxylase and 18-oxidase activities. In the glomerulosa, the CYP11B1 11ß-hydroxylase catalyzes the conversion of desoxycorticosterone (DOC) to corticosterone. The CYP11B2 18-hydroxylase and 18-oxidase activities constitute aldosterone synthase that first converts corticosterone to 18-hydroxycorticosterone (via 18-hydroxylase) and 18-hydroxycorticosterone to aldosterone (via 18-oxidase). CYP11B2 is not normally under ACTH control. CYP11B2 and CYP11B1 are 30 to 40 kb apart.

In GRA, there is a crossover between the two genes, with the 5' portion of the hybrid gene including the CYP11B1 promoter with its ability to respond to ACTH and the 3' portion of the gene including CYP11B2 with its aldosterone synthesis ability. Therefore in GRA, the mutant gene expressed in the fasiculata acquires the ability to produce aldosterone under control of ACTH producing an "ACTH-dependent" hyperaldosteronism. By administering glucocorticoids to suppress endogenous ACTH, the hypertension is abolished because aldosterone production by the fasiculata is suppressed. Because this was initially accomplished with dexamethasone, an older term for GRA is "dexamethasone-suppressible hypertension." While hypokalemia is very common in GRA, some families do not display hypokalemia. Elevated urinary excretion of 18-hydroxy and 18-oxocortisol (steroids not normally found in appreciable amounts) are also observed in GRA. Most GRA families are said to be of Irish lineage.

4) Non-Salt Losing Forms of Congenital Adrenal Hyperplasia

DOC has salt-retaining abilities. Elevated DOC with low aldosterone causes hypertension in 1) two forms of congenital adrenal hyperplasia (CAH): 17α-Hydroxylase deficiency and 11ß-hydroxylase deficiency (Table 5), 2) in cortisol resistance, and 3) in some forms of Cushing syndrome (e.g., ectopic ACTH). DOC can be measured in the serum. Tetrahydroxydesoxycorticosterone is the urinary metabolite of DOC. Cortisol resistance and ectopic ACTH are discussed in the next section.

11ß-Hydroxylase deficiency accounts for ~5% of cases of CAH and results from mutations in the CYP11B1 gene. In brief, deficient 11ß-hydroxylase activity leads to elevated DOC and hypertension onset, usually in childhood. Subsequent to decreased cortisol production, ACTH secretion increases. Elevated ACTH levels drive steroid production in the zona

TABLE 5: COMPARISON OF 17α-HYDROXYLASE DEFICIENT AND 11β-HYDROXYLASE DEFICIENT FORMS OF CAH

	ENZYME DEFICIENCY 17α-HYDROXYLASE	11B-HYDROXYLASE
Gene	CYP17	CYP11B1
17-OHP	Depressed	Elevated
DOC	Elevated	Elevated
Corticosterone	Depressed	Depressed
Desoxycortisol	Depressed	Elevated
Cortisol	Depressed*	Depressed*
17-KGS	Depressed	Elevated
17-OHCS	Depressed	Elevated
17-KS	Depressed	Elevated
Ambiguous genitalia	46XY & 46XX: female phenotype	In females
Precocious puberty	No	In boys
Salt loss	No	No
Hypertension	Late childhood/adolescence	Late childhood/adolescence

* *May be low normal from ACTH stimulation compensating for the metabolic defect.*

glomerulosa and DOC is produced in excess. The high levels of DOC inhibit aldosterone synthase activities and thus aldosterone is not elevated. Because of the metabolic block in cortisol biosynthesis, adrenal steroid production (under the influence of elevated ACTH concentrations) is shifted to adrenal androgen production, leading to elevations in dehydroepiandrosterone (DHEA) and androstenedione. 17-Hydroxyprogesterone is also elevated as the immediate precursor of androstenedione. In female fetuses, exposure to excessive levels of adrenal androgens produces virilization of the external genitalia and ambiguous genitalia. Untreated, girls will virilize further in childhood. Boys with CYP11B1 mutations present with precocious puberty. Infants with this form of CAH do not display salt-losing crises (e.g., Addisonian crisis) because elevated DOC prevents salt wasting. Unless adequately treated with replacement doses of glucocorticoids, "hypokalemic-hypoaldosteronemic" hypertension will develop in children affected with 11ß-hydroxylase deficiency. 11ß-Hydroxylase deficiency leads to elevations in serum desoxycortisol and increased urinary excretion of its metabolite tetrahydrodesoxycortisol (THS).

17α-Hydroxylase deficiency is a rare cause of CAH. Deficiency of this enzyme prevents the conversion of pregnanelone to 17-hydroxypregnanelone and prevents the conversion of progesterone to 17-

hydroxyprogesterone. Therefore there is a severe block in cortisol, adrenal androgen,and sex hormone biosynthesis. CYP17 is the gene that encodes 17α-hydroxylase acitivty in the zona fasiculata. CYP17 mutations will also affect sex steroid production as this gene provides 17,20-desmolase (lyase) activity in the zona reticularis and gonad that converts 17-hydroxypregnanelone to DHEA and 17-hydroxyprogesterone to androstenedione. Therefore CYP17 mutations prevent sex steroid production of both androgens and estrogens. However, the aldosterone pathway is left intact. Similar to 11ß-hydroxylase deficiency, because of cortisol deficiency in 17α-hydroxylase deficiency, ACTH levels rise and drive steroid production in the zona glomerulosa. DOC is produced in excess and high levels of DOC inhibit aldosterone synthesis. Because of the mineralocorticoid activity of DOC, salt-wasting does not occur in 17α-hydroxylase deficiency and hypertension can develop in childhood. Because sex steroids are not produced, 46XY individuals will appear as phenotypic females with delayed puberty. They will lack uterus, fallopian tubes, and the upper 1/3 of the vagina because their testes will produce mullerian inhibiting hormone (also known as anti-mullerian hormone, AMH). However, there is no virilization of the genitalia in utero because of the block in testosterone biosynthesis. In 46XX individuals, there will be no ambiguity of the genitalia; however because estrogens will not be produced, puberty and menses will not occur spontaneously and the patient presents with hypertension, delayed puberty, and amenorrhea.

Besides the phenotypic and clinical distinctions (as discussed above) for 11ß-hydroxylase deficiency and 17α-hydroxylase deficiency, measurement of urinary steroids differentiates these two disorders. 17-KGS, 17-OHCS, and 17-KS are all low in 17α-hydroxylase deficiency. In contrast in untreated 11ß-hydroxylase deficiency, 17-KGS, 17-OHCS, and 17-KS are all elevated.

5) Cortisol Resistance and Ectopic ACTH Cushing Syndrome

Elevated ACTH in cortisol resistance and ectopic ACTH Cushing syndrome also lead to DOC overproduction, salt retention, and hypertension. Cortisol resistance (a very rare syndrome) results from a defect in the glucocorticoid receptor. This defect is also present in hypothalamic and pituitary glucocorticoid receptors. Because cortisol levels are perceived as low because of the glucocorticoid receptor resistance, ACTH levels rise and drive increased cortisol and DOC production. The elevated cortisol levels prevent the development of a clinically hypoglucocorticoid state, yet patients are not usually clinically Cushingoid because of their resistance to cortisol, allowing this condition to be differentiated from Cushing syndrome. However, elevated DOC causes salt retention and hypertension. Elevated ACTH in cortisol resistance can lead to excess adrenal androgen production with hirsutism and pseudoprecocious puberty. A discussion of ectopic ACTH Cushing syndrome is found above.

6) Apparent Mineralocorticoid Excess

In rare cases where hypokalemic hyporeninemic hypertension is associated with depressed aldosterone and DOC, apparent mineralocorticoid excess (AME) should be considered. This rare disorder arises from 11ß-hydroxysteroid dehydrogenase (HSD11B2) deficiency. HSD11B2 normally catalyzes the conversion of cortisol into cortisone in tissues that are normally mineralocorticoid sensitive (e.g, the distal convoluted tubule of the kidney). This conversion also occurs in the liver.

The mineralocorticoid receptor does not distinguish between cortisol and aldosterone. The tissue conversion of cortisol to cortisone protects the mineralocorticoid receptor from cortisol because while cortisol will bind to and activate the mineralocorticoid receptor, cortisone will not. In this way when cortisol is present in normal circulating concentrations, cortisol does not normally stimulate the mineralocorticoid receptor or produce significant mineralocorticoid effects. However with deficiency of HSD11B2, cortisol is not transformed into cortisone in the distal convoluted tubule and cortisol then has mineralocorticoid activity causing salt and water retention that produces hypertension and hypokalemia. HSD11B2 deficiency is diagnosed by an increased ratio of cortisol metabolites to cortisone metabolites [increased ratio of tetrahydrocortisol to tetrahydrocortisone (THF/THE ratio)]. Spironolactone and dexamethasone have been used to treat HSD11B2 deficiency. Incidentally, HSD11B1 (note: not HSD11B2) normally acts to change cortisone into cortisol but is not expressed in tissues that are sensitive to mineralocorticoid. The licorice metabolite glycyrrhetinic acid can inhibit HSD11B2, producing an "acquired" AME syndrome.

III) Pheochromocytoma

A) Clinical Overview

Pheochromocytomas are neuroendocrine tumors that originate predominantly in the adrenal gland medulla. By secreting excessive amounts of catecholamines (e.g., epinephrine, norepinephrine, and/or their precursors or metabolites, Figure 7), pheochromocytomas produce labile or paroxysmal hypertension that is often accompanied by headache, pallor, palpitations, and perspiration. Other clinical findings include nervousness, hypertensive retinopathy, nausea and vomiting, fasting hyperglycemia, hypermetabolism, orthostatic hypotension, and weight loss. In addition to the findings of headaches, tachycardia, and diaphoresis, pheochromocytoma should be considered in patients with a family history of pheochromocytoma, evidence of a multiple endocrine neoplasia syndrome (see Chapter 9), an incidental suprarenal mass, and any history of an adverse cardiovascular response to anesthesia or medications (e.g., opiates, histamine, ACTH, saralasin, and glucagon) known to precipitate symptoms in patients affected with pheochromocytomas.

B) Isolated and Familial Pheochromocytoma

Pheochromocytomas can occur as isolated tumors. However in 5% to 10% of cases, pheochromocytoma occurs as part of an autosomal dominant familial cancer syndrome. Such familial cancer syndromes include multiple endocrine neoplasia types 2A and 2B (see Chapter 9), familial pheochromocytoma syndrome, von Recklinghousen neurofibromatosis type 1, von Hippel-Lindau type II syndrome, tuberous sclerosis, and Sturge-Weber syndrome. Bilateral pheochromocytomas are more common in genetic syndromes because there is an underlying somatic cell mutation in all cells of the body in such conditions. Therefore, only a single additional "hit" (e.g., mutation) is required to trigger the development of a tumor. Whereas only 10% of adults exhibit bilateral pheochromocytomas, 35% of children display bilateral involvement. This likely reflects the fact that genetic syndromes are more common causes of pheochromcytoma in children than in adults. Most pheochromocytomas occur in the fourth and fifth decade of life. Autopsy studies reveal that most pheochromocytomas are not diagnosed premortem.

Five percent of patients with pheochromocytoma have neurofibromatosis. Conversely, 1% of patients with neurofibromatosis develop pheochromocytomas. Neurofibromatosis also includes fibrosarcoma, meningioma, and glioma and results from a mutation in the NF1 gene. Neurofibromin is the protein product of the NF1 locus. At 2818 amino acids with a molecular weigh of 250 kDa, neurofibromin is expressed in brain, spleen, kidney, testis, and thymus. There is functional and structural similarity to GTPase-activating proteins that down-regulate p21-ras which is a cellular proto-oncogene.

Von Hippel-Lindau syndrome, which results from a mutation in the VHL gene, is characterized by cerebellar hemangioblastoma, retinal an-

FIGURE 7. CATECHOLAMINE BIOSYNTHESIS AND DETECTION

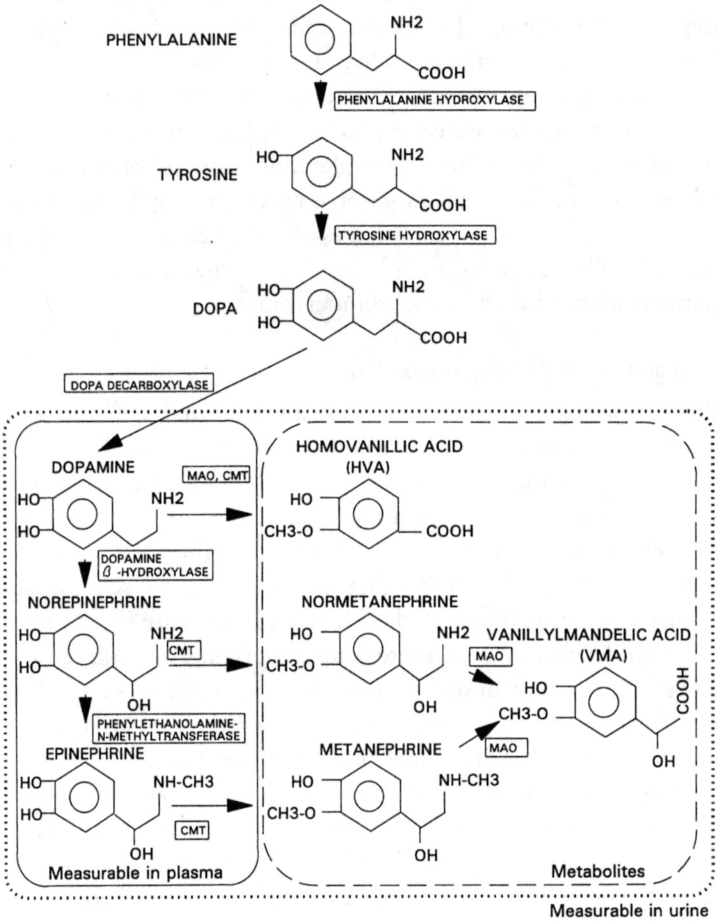

CMT=Catecholamine-O-methyl transerase
MAO=monoamine oxidase

Figure 7: The synthesis of norepinephrine and epinephrine is outlined. Phenylalanine is converted to tyrosine by phenylalanine hydroxylase. Deficiency of this enzyme causes phenylketonuria (PKU). Tyrosine is then hydroxylated to produce dihydroxyphenylalanine (DOPA). Via decarboxylation, dopamine is synthesized. Addition of a hydroxyl group produces norepinephrine whereas further addition of a methyl group to norepinephrine forms epinephrine. Norepinephrine is the normal catecholamine neurotransmitter manufactured in the dendrites of neurons. Epinephrine is the major product of the adrenal medulla whose secretion is controlled by the sympathetic nervous system. HVA is a metabolite of dopamine. The "metanephrines" (see text) are metabolites of norepinephrine and epinephrine. VMA is a metabolite of the metanphrines.

gioma, renal cell carcinomas, and islet cell carcinomas. The VHL gene is located at chromosome 3p25. About 1 in 7 patients with von Hippel-Lindau syndrome will develop a pheochromocytoma. Tuberous sclerosis is characterized by adenoma sebaceum, seizures, and mental deficiency. Capillary and cavernous hemangiomas characterize Sturge-Weber syndrome. Neurofibromatosis, von Hippel-Lindau syndrome, tuberous sclerosis, and Sturge-Weber syndrome are collectively termed neuroectodermal syndromes or phakomatoses.

Most pheochromocytomas are intrabdominal, with <1% located in the neck and 2% to 3% located in the thorax. In the abdomen, up to 80% of pheochromocytomas are located exclusively in the adrenal, whereas 10% are located outside the adrenal (so called "paragangliomas"), and 10% are located both within and outside the adrenal gland. The right adrenal gland is more often affected than the left adrenal gland. Bilateral adrenal pheochromocytomas are found in 5% to 25% of patients. Six to 10% of pheochromocytomas are malignant.

C) Laboratory Diagnosis of the Pheochromocytoma

Biochemically, pheochromocytoma is diagnosed by identification of elevated catecholamine levels in the plasma or urine. Because plasma cat echolamines are extremely variable depending on the state of excitement, stress, and pain that the patient experiences, timed urine collections are usually the preferred samples for analysis. Space does not permit a discussion of imaging techniques for pheochromocytoma, such as abdominal CT or MRI, or [*meta*- ^{125} I]iodobenzylguanidine (MIBG) radionucleotide scanning (scintigraphy). Whereas ~2% of the general population display nonspecific anatomic adrenal abnormalities, radiologic investigation should not be undertaken unless the diagnosis of pheochromocytoma has been established biochemically.

1) Urine Catecholamines

Urine can be collected over a 24 h period for a multiplicity of catecholamine and metabolite assays: dopamine, homovanillic acid (HVA), norepinephrine, epinephrine, metanephrine, normetanephrine, vanillylmandelic acid (VMA), and total catecholamines. The state-of-art assays measure "free" (e.g., unconjugated) catecholamines. "Fractionated" catecholamines usually implies individual measurements of dopamine, norepinephrine, and epinephrine. The terms "metanephrines" and "total metanephrines" are usually used synonymously and represent the sum of the metanephrine plus normetanephrine excretion.

While the choice of analytes measured to diagnose pheochromocytoma varies among endocrinologists, several sources indicate that measurement of norepinephrine, epinephrine, and metanephrines (e.g., total metanephrines) is usually highly effective in detecting elevated catecholamine excretion in pheochromocytoma. Total metanephrines appear to better discriminate pheochromocytoma from other forms of hypertension than measurements of norepinephrine, epinephrine, or VMA. Therefore, total metanephrines appear to be the best single laboratory screening test for pheochromocytoma. As well because of improved methodologies, VMA measurement is generally not required. In pheochromocytoma urinary total metanephrines are usually two- to threefold greater than the upper limit of normal. Higher levels of epinephrine excretion do correlate with an adrenal location of the pheochromocytoma.

Twenty-four hour urines must be acidified (e.g., 25mL of 6N HCl) to stabilize catecholamines and should be assayed for creatinine to assess completeness of collection. Twenty-four hour urine collections for pheochromocytoma screening are superior to spot urine measurements of catecholamine excretion expressed relative to creatinine excretion (mg of catecholamine per g of creatinine). False-positive increases in catecholamines have been observed in patients taking exogenous sympathomimetics, methyldopa, levodopa, and labetalol for up to 2 weeks prior to urinary catecholamine analysis. Metyrosine, reserpine, and guanethidine can falsely depress metanephrine measurements.

2) Plasma Catecholamines

To measure plasma catecholamines, a heparin lock is introduced into a peripheral vein and the patient is allowed to rest in the supine position in a calm environment. Alcohol, caffeine-containing drinks, tobacco, and strenuous exercise should be avoided prior to testing. After 30 minutes, blood is drawn into a wet-ice chilled heparinized (green top) tube and transported to the laboratory on wet ice. The specimen is optimally spun in the cold with the plasma frozen within 15 minutes of collection. Dopamine, norepinephrine, epinephrine, and total catecholamines can be assayed in plasma. The most rigorous plasma catecholamine assays involve HPLC analysis with electrochemical detection. Normally, total catecholamines are <1000 pg/mL. Total catecholamine levels between 1000 and 1999 pg/mL are suggestive of pheochromocytoma, and levels ≥2000 pg/mL are considered to be diagnostic for pheochromocytoma.

The two advantages of measuring plasma epinephrine, norepinephrine, and dopamine are: 1) testing can be performed on a single occasion using a heparin lock, and 2) plasma testing avoids the inconvenience of a timed urine collection. On the other hand, timed urine collections for catecholamines provide an integrated measurement of catecholamine production.

3) Clonidine Suppression Test

In pheochromocytoma, clonidine, a centrally acting α-2 agonist, fails to suppress either plasma or urine catecholamine measurements. Typically, after an overnight fast, 0.3 mg of orally administered clonidine in adults will suppress plasma total catecholamines to ~500 pg/mL. However, in adults with pheochromoctyoma, suppression does not occur. In this test, total catecholamines are measured every 30 minutes for 3 hours following clonidine administration. Antihypertensives (excluding α1-blockers such as phenoxybenzamine and phentolamine) should be discontinued for ≥2 days before testing.

4) Sequential Testing

A sequential approach to testing would include the following steps. 1) Measurement of a 24 hr urine collection for norepinephrine, epinephrine, and metanephrines. 2) If the results of the urine studies are equivocal, measure plasma catecholamines. 3) If the plasma catecholamine results are equivocal, repeat the measurements before and after clonidine. 4) If these results are still equivocal, consider chromogranin A measurement or repeat urine evaluations. Chromogranin A is not specific for pheochromocytoma but serum concentrations may be elevated up to tenfold greater than in other forms of hypertension. Measuring platelet catecholamine concentrations does not appear to be advantagous over other forms of testing for pheochromocytoma and displays a high false-positive frequency.

A clinical history consistent with pheochromocytoma associated with elevated plasma or urine catecholamine concentrations should then trigger a radiographic workup for pheochromocytoma. The definitive therapy for pheochromocytoma is surgical removal.

References

1. Graybeal ML, Fang VS. Physiological dosing of exogenous ACTH. Acta Endocrin 1985;108:401-406.
2. Jones KL. The Cushing syndromes. Pediatr Clin North Am 1990;37:1313-1332.
3. Carey RM, Varma SK, Drake CR, Thorner MO, Kovacs K, Ribier J,

Vale W. Ectopic secretion of corticotropin-releasing factor as a cause of Cushing syndrome. N Engl J Med 1984;311:13-20.

4. Oldfield EH, Doppman JL, Nieman LK, Chrousos GP, Miller DL, Katz DA, Cutler GB, Loriaux LL. Petrosal venous sampling with and without corticotropin-releasing hormone for the differntial diagnosis of Cushing syndrome. N Engl J Med 1991;325:897-905.
5. Tabarin A, Greselle JF, San-Balli F, Leprat F, Caille JM, Latapie JL, Guerin J, Roger P. Usefulness of the corticotropin-releasing hormone test during bilateral inferior petrosal sinus sampling for the diagnosis of Cushing syndrome. J Clin Endo Metabol 1991;73:53-59.
6. Yanovski JA, Cutler GB, Doppman JL, Miller DL, Chrousos GP, Oldfield EH, Nieman LK. The limited ability of inferior pertrosal sinus sampling with corticotropin-releasing hormone to distinguish Cushing disease from pseudo-Cushing states or normal physiology. J Clin Endo Metabol 1992;77:503-509.

General References

1. Granner DK. Hormones of the Adrenal Cortex. In: Murray RK, Granner DK, Mayes PA, Rodwell VW eds. Harper's Biochemistry 22nd ed. Norwalk: Appleton & Lange, 1990:499-510.
2. Migeon CJ, Donohoue P. Adrenal Disorders. In: Kappy MS, Blizzard RM, Migeon CJ eds. Wilkin's-The Diagnosis and Treatment of Endocrine Disorders in Childhood and Adolescence, 4th ed. Springfield, Il: Charles C. Thomas Co. Publishers, 1994:717-856.
3. Orth DN, Kovacs WJ, DeBold CR. The Adenal Cortex. In: Wilson JD, Foster DW eds. Williams Textbook of Endocrinology, 8th ed. Philadelphia: WB Saunders, 1992:489-620.
4. Whitley RJ, Meikle AW, Watts NB. Adrenocortical steroids. In: Burtis CA, Ashwood ER, eds. Tietz Textbook of Clinical Chemistry 2nd ed. Philadelphia: WB Saunders, 1994:1796-1843.
5. Williams GH, Dluhy RG. Diseases of the Adrenal Cortex. In: Wilson JD, Braunwald E, Isselbacher KJ, Petersdorf RG, Fauci AS, Root RK eds. Harrison's Principles of Internal Medicine, 12th ed. New York: McGraw-Hill, 1991:1713-1734.
6. White PC. Disorders of aldosterone biosynthesis and action. N Engl J Med 1994;331:250-258.
7. Krohn K, Uibo R, Aavik E, Peterson P, Savilahti K. Identification by molecular cloning of an autoantigen associated with Addison's dis-

ease as steroid 17 alpha-hydroxylase. Lancet 1992;339:770-773.

8. Baumann-Antczak A, Wedlock N, Bednarek J, Kiso Y, Krishnan H, Fowler S, Smith BR, Furmaniak J. Autoimmune Addison's disease and 21-hydroxylase. Lancet 1992;340:429-430.

9. Winqvist O, Gustafsson J, Rorsman F, Karlsson FA, Kämpe O. Two different cytochrome P450 enzymes are the adrenal antigens in autoimmune polyendocrine syndrome type I and Addison's disease. J Clin Invest 1993;92:2377-2385.

10. Neufeld M, Maclaren N, Blizzard R. Autoimmune polyglandular syndromes. Pediatr Ann 1980;9:43-53.

11. White PC, New MI, Dupont B. Congenital adrenal hyperplasia, part 1. N Engl J Med 1987;316(24):1519-1524.

12. White PC, New MI, Dupont B. Congenital adrenal hyperplasia, part 2. N Engl J Med 1987;316(25):1580-1586.

13. Miller WL, Levine LS. Molecular and clinical advances in congenital adrenal hyperplasia. J Pediatr 1987;111(1):1-17.

14. Ketchum C, Riley WJ, Maclaren NK. Adrenal dysfunction in asymptomatic patients with adrenocortical autoantibodies. J Clin Endo Metab 1984;58:1166-1170.

15. Trainer PJ, McAhrdy KC, Reid IW. Urinary free cortisol in the assessment of hydrocortisone replacement therapy. Horm Metab Res 1993;25:117-120.

16. Roccella EJ; Update on the 1987 Task Force Report on High Blood Pressure in Children and Adolescents: A Working Group Report from the National BP Education Program: Pediatrics 1986; 98(4):649-58.

17. Laragh JH, Letcher RL, Pickering TG: Renin Profiling for diagnosis and treatment of hypertension. JAMA 1979; 241:151-56.

18. Bravo EL, Tarazi RC, Fouad FM, Vidt DG, Gifford RW. Clonidine-suppression test, a useful aid in the diagnosis of pheochromocytoma. N Engl J Med 1981; 305:623-626.

19. Muller FB, Sealey JE, Case DB, et al.: The Captopril test for identifying renvascular disease in hypertensive patients. American Journal of Med. 1986: 633-44.

20. Rosano TG, Swift TA, Hayes LW: Advances in catecholamine and metabolite measurements for diagnosis of pheochromocytoma. Clin Chem 1991;37/10(B):1854-67.

21. Sealey JE: Plasma renin activity and plasma prorenin assays. Clin. Chem. 1991; 37/10(B): 1811-19.
22. Bravo EL, Grifford RW, and Manger WM. Adrenal Medullary Tumors Pheochromocytoma: In Mazzaferri EL, Samaan NA, eds. Endocrine Tumors. ; Boston:Blackwell Scientific Publications, Inc.; 1993: p. 426-47.
23. Scully RE, Mark EJ, McNeely WF, McNeely BU : Case records of the massachusetts general hospital.; weekly clinicopathological exercises. N Engl J Med 1992: 326 (24):1617-1623.
24. Gerlo EAM, Sevens C: Urinary and plasma catecholamines and urinary catecholamine metabolites in pheochromocytoma: diagnositic value in 19 cases. Clin Chem 1994; 40:250-256.
25. The Sixth Report of the Joint National Committee on Prevention, Detection, Evaluation, and Treatment of High Blood Pressure. Arch Intern Med 1997;157:2413-46.
26. Dons RF, editor. Endocrine and Metabolic Testing Manual 3rd ed. Boca Raton,: CRC Press LLC; 1998.
27. Orth DN: Cushing syndrome. N Engl J Med 1994; 332:791-803.

4
Endocrine Disorders of the Reproductive System

LAURENCE M. DEMERS, PHD, DABCC

The process and control of reproduction in the human species involves an intricate and complex integration of hormonal signals that starts in the hypothalamic region of the brain and transcends through the pituitary gland to the reproductive organs, where hormonal products produced by the gonads feedback to control the entire process of hormone secretion. The regulation of gonadotropin secretion starts in the hypothalamus with the pulsatile release of gonadotropin-releasing hormone (GnRH). GnRH travels by way of the portal circulation to the pituitary and through a conventional receptor-cell signaling activation process that involves G-proteins linked to adenylate cyclase, gonadotropin-producing cells are activated to synthesize and secrete follicle-stimulating hormone (FSH) and luteinizing hormone (LH) in a similar pulsatile fashion. FSH then acts as a trophic and gametogenic hormone to both the ovary and testes and stimulates the maturation of ovarian follicles in the female and promotes the process of spermatogenesis in the testes of the male. The mechanism of action of LH on the other hand on both the ovary and testes is to facilitate steroidogenesis. The synthesis and release of estradiol and progesterone from the ovary in the female and testosterone synthesis by the testes in the male come under the direct effect of LH.

Regulation of Gn-RH and Gonadotropin Secretion

The negative feedback loop so characteristic in endocrinology is an important feature in the regulatory control of the hypothalamic-pituitary-gonadal axis. In the male, the testes produces two important products that govern the negative feedback response to higher centers of control in the brain: inhibin and testosterone. Inhibin is a protein made by Sertoli cells of the testes that negatively feed back at the level of the pituitary to control the synthesis and release of FSH. In contrast, testosterone made by Leydig cells in the testes elicits negative feedback control for FSH and LH at both the level of the hypothalamus and pituitary. In the female, the negative feedback loop between the ovary and the brain is a bit more complex than in the male. Estrogen released from the ovary exerts both a positive and a negative feedback effect on gonadotropin secretion at the level of the hypothalamus and pituitary depending on the time of the reproductive cycle and the concentration and duration of exposure to the steroid. Estrogen is inhibitory to both FSH and LH secretion at both low and high concentrations over a specific period of time within the normal menstrual cycle, with one exception. At the time of ovulation in the menstrual cycle, a sharp rise in estrogen release from the ovary triggers gonadotropin secretion. This results in a surge of LH secretion that initiates the process of ovulation. Progesterone has an inhibitory effect on Gn-RH secretion at the level of the hypothalamus. Inhibin made by granulosa cells in the ovary also plays a negative feedback role in FSH secretion at the level of the pituitary.

Chemistry and Function of the Gonadotropins

Both FSH and LH are glycoproteins that exists as heterodimers and have a strong sequence homology to other pituitary hormones. TSH and human chorionic gonadotropin share α-subunit sequence homology with both FSH and LH. The specificity of the gonadotropins resides in their unique amino acid sequence of the β-subunit and the degree of glycosylation found in this subunit. The actions of gonadotropins are confined to the ovary and testis.

In the female, FSH promotes growth and maturation of the developing ovarian follicles, stimulates the appearance of ovarian LH receptors, and facilitates the aromatization of androgens to estrogens. LH, on the other hand, promotes ovarian steroidogenesis, induces ovulation and rupture of the mature follicle and maintains the corpus luteum and progesterone secretion.

In the male, FSH is responsible for spermatogenesis, induction of Leydig cell maturation, stimulation of androgen binding protein and induction of LH receptors on Leydig cells. LH, on the other hand, promotes testosterone biosynthesis from the testes.

Female Reproductive Disorders

Disorders of the hypothalamic-pituitary gonadal axis can present at any age and are usually categorized into two major classifications in reproductive age women; primary ovarian failure leading to hypergonadotropic hypogonadism and dysfunction of the hypothalamic-pituitary axis leading to hypogonadotropic hypogonadism or secondary ovarian failure. (Table 1) Endocrine disorders in the prepubertal years are a category of their own. Any pathologic elevation in FSH and LH is usually indicative of primary gonadal failure and can be caused by a variety of abnormalities ranging from defects in ovarian steroidogenesis to premature ovarian failure caused by radiation injury or autoimmune diseases. Table 1 list the major categories of primary and secondary ovarian failure that occur in reproductive age women. At the time of menopause, the ovaries senesce, resulting in a decline in both inhibin and steroid production and a hypergonadotropic response. A rise in FSH occurs first in women entering menopause as a result of the decline in inhibin production. This event is followed later by a rise in LH as ovarian steroidogenesis decreases.

Hypogonadotropic disorders in females are due to diseases that affect either the hypothalamus, pituitary or a combination of both. In these patients a loss in cyclical gonadal function occurs if menstrual cycles existed prior to the disease onset. Diseases of the hypothalamus which result in deficient Gn-RH production include brain tumors, infections such as tuberculosis and meningitis and a disorder called hypothalamic amenorrhea in which a pulsatile defect in the Gn-RH pulse generator occurs in patients who have malnutrition or have endured excessive strenuous exercise. Pituitary causes of deficient gonadotropin production include pituitary tumors, pituitary necrosis as a result of an infarction and pituitary inflammatory diseases such as sarcoidosis or hemochromatosis.

Table 1. Female Reproductive Disorders

I. Hypergonadotropic Hypogonadism

A. Gonadal Agenesis

B. Gonadal Dysgenesis

- 1. Abnormal karyotype
  - a. Turner's syndrome, 45X
  - b. Mosaicism
- 2. Normal karyotype
  - a. Pure gonadal dysgenesis

C. Ovarian Steroidogenesis Defect

- 1. 17α-hydroxylase deficiency
- 2. 17,20-lyase deficiency

D. Premature Ovarian Failure

- 1. Injury
  - a. Mumps oophoritis
  - b. Radiation
  - c. Chemotherapy
- 2. Resistant ovary syndrome
- 3. Autoimmune disease

E. Chronic Anovulation

- 1. PCOS
- 2. Adrenal disease
  - a. Cushing
  - b. Adrenal hyperplasia
- 3. Thyroid disease
- 4. Ovarian tumor

II. Hypogonadotropic Hypogonadism

A. Hypothalamus

- 1. Tumors
- 2. Infection
  - a. Tuberculosis
  - b. Syphilis
  - c. Meningitis
  - d. Sarcoidosis
- 3. Functional Gn-RH defect
  - a. Chronic stress
  - b. Malnutrition
  - c. Strenuous exercise
  - d. Kallmanns syndrome

B. Pituitary

- 1. Adenoma
- 2. Necrosis
  - a. Sheehan's syndrome
  - b. Panhypopituitarism
- 3. Inflammatory disorders
  - a. Sarcoidosis
  - b. Hemochromatosis

Prepubertal disorders

Precocious puberty is a prepubertal disorder that is ten times more common in girls than boys. Sometimes call isosexual precocity, idiopathic precocious puberty is responsible for over 90% of the cases where no identifiable cause for premature maturation of the hypothalamic-pituitary axis can be found. The remaining 10% of cases are due to tumors of the central nervous system. The diagnosis is made by exclusion. Basal levels of the gonadotropins and gonadal steroids are increased to adult levels and the expression of secondary sex characteristics can be quite striking. Short stature can be a common physical consequence of precocious puberty. If left undiagnosed, precocious puberty can result in considerable emotional and psychological problems.

Male reproductive disorders

Gonadal disorders in the male usually present as either hypergonadotropic hypogonadism or hypogonadotropic hypogonadism. (Table 2) In the former, the hypothalamic-pituitary axis is intact and primary gonadal disease leads to a loss in negative feedback control, resulting in significant, unregulated increases in gonadotropin production.

Hypergonadotropic Hypogonadism. There are many causes of primary gonadal failure, ranging from a developmental defect in testicular growth, as observed with complete gonadal agenesis, to mild testicular injury that results from either a viral infection, radiation injury or other causes. The most common testicular developmental defect is Klinefelter's syndrome. This is a chromosomal abnormality (47,XXY) that afflicts one in 500 males and is associated with dysgenesis of the seminiferous tubules, a lack of sperm production and marked elevations in FSH. Other genetic abnormalities that result in primary gonadal failure include 46,XY/XXY mosaicism, the XX male syndrome and Noonan's syndrome. Noonan's syndrome is an autosomal dominant disorder with clinical expressions of short stature, webbed neck, cryptorchidism and mental retardation. This disorder parallels the unusual features found in Turner's syndrome in girls.

Primary testicular failure can result from direct injury to the testes. Mumps orchitis, granulomatous diseases, autoimmune disease, radiation injury and medications associated with chemotherapy can damage the testes and produce an inability to make sperm or synthesize the sex steroid testosterone. Select damage to the testes can result in a situation in which testosterone production may be normal but spermatogenesis is

Table 2. Male Reproductive Disorders

I. Hypergonadotropic hypogonadism

A. Gonadal agenesis

B. Gonadal dysgenesis

- 1. Abnormal karyotype
  - a. Klinefelters Syndrome
  - b. XX male syndrome

C. Testicular Failure

- 1. Injury
  - a. Viral orchitis
  - b. Trauma
  - c. Radiation
  - d. Chemotherapy
  - e. Drugs (Spironolactone)
- 2. Autoimmune disease
- 3. Granulomatous disease
- 4. Androgen resistance syndrome
- 5. Germinal cell aplasia
- 6. Cryptorchidism
- 7. Varicocele
- 8. Immotile cilia syndrome
- 9. Germ cell tumors

D. Chronic disease

- 1. Liver disease
- 2. Renal failure
- 3. Neurological disease
- 4. Sickle cell anemia

II. Hypogonadotropic Hypogonadism

A. Hypothalamus

- 1. Tumors
- 2. Infection
  - a. Tuberculosis
  - b. Syphilis
  - c. Meningitis
  - d. Sarcoidosis
- 3. Functional GN-RH defect
  - a. Chronic Stress
  - b. Malnutrition
  - c. Strenuous exercise
  - d. Kallmanns syndrome

B. Pituitary

- 1. Adenoma
- 2. Inflammatory disorder
  - a. Sarcoidosis
  - b. Hemochromatosis
- 3. Isolated FSH deficiency

impaired. In this case, FSH levels are raised but LH levels remain relatively normal. This is the usual pattern seen in patients who develop viral induced orchitis in which damage to the seminiferous tubules occur and yet Leydig cells are not affected. Testicular injury as a result of chemotherapy can be quite common in male cancer patients and can lead to permanent testicular damage and gonadal failure.

While testicular failure is the most common cause of hypergonadotropic hypogonadism, overproduction of gonadotropins can occur in patients with gonadotropin-secreting pituitary tumors. These patients typically secrete large amounts of inactive subunits which do not bind to gonadotropin receptors in the testes but give the biochemical appearance of increased gonadotropin levels.

Hypogonadotropic hypogonadism. This disorder results from a disruption in the normal signaling events in the hypothalamic-pituitary-gonadal axis due to either a deficiency or dysregulation in the pulsatile secretion of Gn-RH from the hypothalamus or as a result of a pituitary defect in gonadotropin synthesis and/or secretion. Chromosomal abnormalities account for a significant portion of those disorders associated with abnormal synthesis of Gn-RH. Kallmann's syndrome is an X-linked disorder characterized by isolated deficiency in Gn-RH secretion in the absence of any demonstrated CNS lesion. Besides hypogonadism, this disorder is associated with a variety of somatic defects including a decrease or complete absence of olfactory sense, deafness, a tendency toward cleft palate and color blindness. If diagnosed properly, this disorder can be treated by the exogenous administration of Gn-RH given in a pulsatile mode. Other causes of a compromise in pulsatile hypothalamic Gn-RH release include brain tumors such as a craniopharyngioma or glioma, radiation to the head and neck region and infiltrative disorders of the hypothalamus including histiocytosis and sarcoid. Recently it has been shown that extreme strenuous exercise can produce a pulsatile defect in the secretion of Gn-RH that results in a hypogonadotropic response. Strenuous exercise such as long distance running can provoke a dysregulation in the GnRH pulse generator, resulting in inappropriate gonadotropin release and transient hypogonadism. This can occur in both men and women, although it is more common in women.

Pituitary causes of hypogonadotropism are relatively rare in men but can occur. Men with prolactin secreting pituitary adenomas, acromegaly, hypothyroidism, pituitary infarction, empty sella syndrome, sarcoidosis, and hemochromatosis can develop hypogonadotropic hypogonadism. Unlike anorexia nervosa and its prevalence in the female population, nutritional deficiency is a rare cause of gonadotropin deficiency in males. Renal failure can be a cause of a functional hypothalamic-pituitary disorder and must be considered in the differential diagnosis of hypogonadotropic hypogonadism.

True precocious puberty can also occur in males although less frequently than in females. These children have premature activation of the LH-RH pulse generator resulting in increased synthesis of LH. The rise in LH results in increased secretion of gonadal steroids and the appearance of premature secondary sex characteristics including phallic enlargement, facial and pubic hair, atypical skeletal growth and maturation and other signs and symptoms of androgens. Although the typical age for the onset of precocious puberty is 6 to 7 years, about 25% of children will present with adult testosterone levels and precocious puberty in the 2 to 6 year age bracket. Causes of precocious puberty include CNS tumors, head trauma, infections, radiation to the head and congenital adrenal hyperplasia.

Laboratory Diagnosis of Reproductive Disorders

The complex nature of the hypothalamic-pituitary-axis in both the male and the female make the diagnosis of reproductive disorders an inexact science. Disorders in the reproductive-age female are easier to expose because menstrual cycle disturbances with resulting amenorrhea are an early outward sign that dysfunction of the hypothalamic-pituitary-gonadal-axis may be present. In the adult male, it is more difficult to diagnose a reproductive disorder since unlike the female who has the monthly appearance of menses to reflect the intactness of the hypothalamic-pituitary-gonadal-axis, males do not possess an overt sign of an endocrine disturbance and tend to present much later in the disease than females. The development of a prolactinoma is a prime example of this point. Males tend to initially present with a much larger prolactin secreting macroadenoma of the pituitary compared to females who usually present earlier with a microadenoma. Changes in libido are usually the first outward sign that an endocrine abnormality exists in the adult male regardless of the type of reproductive disorder manifested. However, prepubertal disorders in both sexes can and do present in mild forms and it sometimes takes the expertise of a pediatric endocrinologist to sort out the endocrine disorder. Endocrine reproductive disorders are obviously not a major problem in the postmenopausal female but continue to be a consideration in the elderly male. A low testosterone output can affect the quality of life in males well into the eighth and ninth decades of life.

The laboratory approach to the diagnosis of a reproductive disorder in the reproductive-age female can be categorized into two general areas, infertility and hirsutism. In the adult male. Infertility and decreased libido are the two principal reproductive disorders that bring them to seek medical attention.

Evaluation of the Adult Male

Infertility

Semen analysis and testing the integrity of the hypothalamic-pituitary-testicular axis by measuring serum testosterone and gonadotropin levels (FSH and LH) are the usual approach for assessing the fertility status of the male.

Semen Analysis. Following the procurement of a semen sample by ejaculation, the specimen is usually analyzed for volume, sperm count, sperm morphology, motility and the presence of fructose. Results are compared to normalized values from healthy male donors.

Basal serum gonadotropin and testosterone levels. Basal serum levels of total testosterone, FSH and LH are determined using specific immunoassay methods. Results are compared to normal reference values from a healthy male population. In most laboratories, the reference range for total serum testosterone falls between 250 - 1,000 ng/dL, while serum FSH and LH values are usually less than 15 mIU/ml.

Interpretation: Males with true primary hypogonadism will have total testosterone values below 200 ng/dl and FSH and LH values greater than 20 mIU/ml. Patients with true hypogonadotropic hypogonadism will have total testosterone values less than 150 ng/dL and gonadotropin values less than 10 mIU/ml.

Urine gonadotropin levels. the pulsatile nature of gonadotropin secretion can frequently produce undetectable serum FSH and LH levels in normal males depending on when the sample is collected. To facilitate the interpretation of low gonadotropin levels in both adult males and in prepubertal males, two approaches can be taken. 1) Collect 3 individual blood samples for serum FSH and LH over a one-hour period. The samples are then pooled and run as a single specimen to integrate the pulsatility. 2) Collect a timed urine sample over the course of three hours and determine the urine level of FSH and LH in that specimen. The urine gonadotropin assays have the advantage that they integrate the pulsatility in pituitary gonadotropin secretion over the three-hour period and allow for concentration of the urine sample. This leads to detectable gonadotropin levels at the low end in the adult male and to measurable levels in prepubertal children.

Note: It is important to recognize that a circadian rhythm in the daily secretion of testosterone also occurs with higher blood levels of testosterone in the morning time period (7-10 AM) when compared to samples collected in the afternoon and evening (> 3 PM). Most laboratories establish their reference values using AM specimens; thus it is recommended that AM collections for testosterone be obtained. It is not uncommon for the same patient to have an abnormally low testosterone level from a clinic sample taken at 4 PM on one day and a normal testosterone level collected at 9 AM the following day.

HCG stimulation test. Males with borderline or suppressed total testosterone values can be evaluated with an hCG stimulation test. hCG binds to LH receptors in the normal testes and stimulates testosterone production. Following the collection of a basal AM testosterone sample, 5,000 units of hCG are administered intramuscularly and a serum testosterone level obtained three days later.

Interpretation: A doubling of the testosterone value from baseline is consistent with normal Leydig cell function. Failure to elevate testosterone by at least 150 ng/dL is indicative of testicular failure and primary hypogonadism.

Gn-RH stimulation test. Patients with hypogonadotropic hypogonadism can be tested by the administration of exogenous Gn-RH to distinguish hypothalamic dysfunction from pituitary disease. Because the pituitary is sensitive to sex steroids for appropriate gonadotropin secretion, patients with long-standing functional hypogonadism must be given exogenous testosterone for at least one week prior to performing the Gn-RH stimulation test. To perform the test, patients are given 100 μg of synthetic Gn-RH intravenously and blood for FSH and LH is collected at baseline and again at 30, 60, 120 and 180 minutes after the infusion of Gn-RH.

Interpretation: An increase in serum gonadotropins of at least 10 mIU/ml from baseline is observed in normal individuals. Patients with pituitary disease will demonstrate little or no rise in the gonadotropins while patients with hypothalamic disease will demonstrate a delayed but significant rise of at least 7 mIU/ml in serum FSH and/or LH within 180 minutes of the infusion of Gn-RH.

Clomiphene stimulation test. Testing of the hypothalamic-pituitary reserve can be achieved with clomiphene, a drug that has anti-estrogenic effects and triggers the activation of Gn-RH secretion by the hypothalamus by blocking the negative feedback effect of estradiol. Inhibition of estradiol in both males and females induces activation of the Gn-RH pulse mechanism which in turn stimulates the secretion of FSH and LH by the pituitary. Baseline blood levels of FSH, LH and testosterone are obtained just prior to the oral administration of 100 mg clomiphene and again at 3 and 7 days after the start of daily clomiphene treatment.

Interpretation: Normal individuals will show a rise in both FSH and LH of greater than 20 mIU/ml within 7 days following the daily administration of clomiphene. A blunted response is observed in patients with an abnormal Gn-RH pulse mechanism due to hypothalamic disease, anorexia nervosa, strenuous exercise, and hyperprolactinemia. Patients with other pituitary diseases and prepubertal children will also show a decreased response.

Evaluation of the prepubertal male

The assessment of the prepubertal male for the most part takes place under two circumstances; precocious puberty and delayed onset of puberty. In precocious puberty, the physical manifestation of androgen excess along with the measurement of testosterone and the gonadotropins can usually help establish the diagnosis. If congenital adrenal hyperplasia (CAH) due to a steroidogenic enzyme defect is the cause of the androgen excess, steroid measurements of adrenal origin are necessary to confirm the disorder. Determination of the adrenal steroids 17α-hydroxyprogesterone and 11β-deoxycortisol helps establish the diagnosis of congenital adrenal hyperplasia and a deficiency in either 21- or 11-hydroxylase enzyme activity respectively. These two enzyme defects are the two most common causes of congenital adrenal hyperplasia.

The measurement of steroids from the adrenal androgen pathway is useful in both documenting the presence of CAH and to follow steroid replacement therapy. Dehydroepiandrosterone (DHEA) and its sulfate derivative and androstenedione are the principal steroids that reflect the adrenal androgen pathway. The secretion of adrenal androgens typically falls under the control of ACTH. With CAH, they are formed in excess as a result of enzyme defects in the cortisol biosynthetic pathway and a diversion of precursor steroids into the adrenal androgen pathway as a result of a compensatory rise in ACTH.

Constitutional delay of puberty (i.e. delayed onset of maturity) is a common presentation in males and establishing normality of the hypothalamic-pituitary-gonadal axis in these patients is helpful to differentiate constitutional delay from true hypogonadism. In the prepubertal years, circulating gonadotropin levels and testosterone are low. With the onset of puberty, the pulsatile secretion of gonadotropins increases in a stepwise fashion and brings about testicular enlargement, spermatogenesis and testosterone production. The timing of puberty appears to be genetically programmed and in some families males may not reach full puberty until the age of 16 years. Because constitutional delay in puberty is a relatively common event and yet can be confused clinically with hypogonadotropic hypogonadism, it becomes important to distinguish the two because there is hormonal treatment available for the latter.

Urine gonadotropin measurements have been shown to be of use in helping make the distinction between true hypogonadotropic hypogonadism and constitutional delay of puberty. Pediatric endocrinologists have used urinary gonadotropin results to distinguish the two and have come to rely on the slope of the line that depicts the linear increase in gonadotropin secretion that occurs normally over several months during progression through puberty. Timed urine gonadotropin measurements are also easy to perform repeatedly in children and the integration of gonadotropin pulsatility and the ability to concentrate the urine allows for appropriate detection of gonadotropins in prepubertal children as well as in pubertal males and females.

Evaluation of the adult female

As mentioned previously, two principal categories comprise the vast majority of female patients who present to their obstetrician with reproductive disorders that require a laboratory workup: infertility and hirsutism. Hirsutism is relatively straightforward and can range from mild clinical manifestations of increased facial and body hair with acne to an overt presentation of hyperandrogenism with severe cystic acne, significant amounts of body hair, clitoromegaly, amenorrhea and a deepening voice. The latter is frequently associated with patients who have an ovarian or adrenal tumor that is hypersecreting androgens.

The presence of amenorrhea and infertility can be a complicated disorder in the reproductive age female and could involve dysfunction at multiple points in the hypothalamic-pituitary-ovarian axis.

Infertility

Pituitary function testing is the first target for the obstetrician when evaluating menstrual irregularities and causes for infertility. Ruling out a treatable reproductive abnormality is the first step for the patient desiring to conceive. An inability to have children as a result of an anatomic abnormality or hormonal problems however is no longer a foregone conclusion since assisted reproductive technologies are readily available and can now result in a healthy pregnancy in many women unable to conceive normally and who wish to bear their own children.

Basal gonadotropin levels. The measurement of FSH and LH in blood or urine helps establish whether the dynamics of the hypothalamic-pituitary-ovarian axis are intact. Because of the pulsatile nature of gonadotropin secretion, a single blood sample for either FSH or LH is difficult to interpret when assessing adequacy of gonadotropin production. A 2-3 fold difference in LH levels for example can be seen in the same individual as a result of simply collecting the blood samples 40 minutes apart. As previously mentioned with males, two approaches are used to assess appropriateness of FSH and LH secretion. Either the collection of 3 blood samples over a one-hour time period and pooling aliquots to analyze as one sample or the use of a timed urine sample over the course of three hours will accurately reflect appropriateness of gonadotropin secretion.

Interpretation: Normal circulating levels of the gonadotropins depend on the time of the menstrual cycle. In general, blood FSH levels are less than 17 mIU/ml during the follicular phase of the menstrual cycle and less than 12 mIU/ml during the luteal phase. Blood LH levels are less than 30 mIU/ml in the follicular phase and less than 20 mIU/ml in the luteal phase. Urine FSH levels range from 120 to 1,490 mIU/hr in reproductive age women while LH values range from 190 to 3,350 mIU/hr in this same population. Females with hypogonadotropic hypogonadism will have undetectable blood levels of FSH and LH and urine levels in the 10 - 100 mIU/hr range. Females with hypergonadotropic hypogonadism from either a regulatory dysfunction or menopause will have blood FSH and LH levels in excess of 40 mIU/ml.

Gonadotropin-Releasing Hormone Stimulation Test (Gn-RH stimulation test). To determine if the defect in gonadotropin secretion resides in the hypothalamus or in the pituitary, a Gn-RH stimulation test can be used to directly stimulate the pituitary. As in the male, the female pituitary is sensitive to sex steroid exposure and therefore it is important in patients with long standing gonadal failure to sensitize the patient by administering estradiol at least one week prior to performing the Gn-RH stimulation test. To perform the test, 100 ug Gn-RH is administered intravenously following baseline collection of blood for FSH, LH and estradiol. Additional blood samples for FSH and LH are taken at 30, 60, 120 and 180 minutes after Gn-RH administration.

Interpretation: A normal response is observed when gonadotropin levels increase over baseline by at least 7 mIU/ml. Patients with a pituitary defect will show little or no rise in gonadotropins while women with hypothalamic disease will show a delay in the rise of gonadotropins but a significant elevation in both FSH and LH of at least 5 mIU/ml within 180 minutes after Gn-RH administration.

Clomiphene stimulation test. Another means of testing the hypothalamic-pituitary reserve is the clomiphene simulation test. This is a functional test that uses the drug clomiphene, which has anti-estrogenic properties and triggers activation of the Gn-RH pulse generator by blocking the effects of endogenous estrogen. Estradiol is normally inhibitory to the hypothalamic Gn-RH secretory mechanism. Antagonism of the estrogen effect will elicit a bolus release of Gn-RH and produce increased pituitary secretion of FSH and LH. The test is performed by giving the patient 100 mg of an oral dose of clomiphene after baseline levels of estradiol, FSH and LH have been obtained. Clomiphene is administered daily for 5 days and additional blood samples for FSH, LH and estradiol are taken 5, 7, 10, 13 and 21 days after the start of the test.

Interpretation: A rise in blood FSH to at least 20 mIU/ml and an increase in LH to at least 30 mIU/ml will occur with clomiphene administration in normal individuals. Patients with a pulsatile defect in Gn-RH secretion due to hypothalamic disease will show a blunted response. In addition, patients with pituitary tumors and anorexia nervosa will also show a reduced response. A pulsatile defect in the Gn-RH pulse generator has been demonstrated in women who exercise strenuously and to excess. This defect for example, has been observed in women who are long distance runners. The excessive strenuous exercise that accompanies long distance running can lead to the disorder termed "jogger's amenorrhea." In these women, amenorrhea is particularly prevalent during the summer months and normal menstrual cyclicity returns in the winter when running frequency is reduced.

The clomiphene stimulation test can also be used to test for luteal phase deficiency. Collection of a blood sample for progesterone on day 21 of the clomiphene stimulation test can be used to document inadequate luteinization in patients with persistent infertility. A normal progesterone level on day 21 would suggest normal luteal function.

Hirsutism

Hirsutism is a common clinical manifestation in women that is associated with relatively benign but annoying symptoms such as excessive facial hair and mild manifestations of virilization. Hirsutism, however, can also be associated with other more significant abnormalities, such as polycystic ovarian disease and tumors of the ovary and adrenal. The virilizing symptoms are associated with excessive production and availability of androgens. Thus it is important for obstetricians and endocrinologists to screen for androgen excess because androgen producing tumors not only cause infertility but can be life threatening and are a resectable curable lesion if diagnosed early enough.

Evaluation of patients with hirsutism. The measurement of androgens in the blood provides a good screening tool to determine whether an androgen excess state exist and whether the levels suggest the presence of either an ovarian or adrenal tumor. Total testosterone as well as free and albumin bound testosterone (bioavailable testosterone) and DHEA-S levels are good screening tests to determine the presence of androgen over production. If any of the above steroid test results are abnormal, it is sometimes useful to measure additional steroids including androstenedione and cortisol to sort out the source of the increased steroid level. Measurement of 3α-androstanediol glucuronide, a tissue metabolite of dihydrotestosterone, is sometimes used to determine whether excessive androgen metabolism is originating in the pilosebaceous unit of the skin.

The absolute levels of total testosterone as well as the mass of free and albumin-bound testosterone along with DHEA-S help define the degree of androgen excess and determine whether further testing is necessary. The upper limit of normal for total testosterone levels in the female is 80 ng/dl. In patients with androgen excess, the percentage and level of free and albumin bound testosterone are also elevated. Measurements of bioavailable testosterone (in contrast to measuring just free testosterone) are preferred by endocrinologists because bioavailable testosterone reflects albumin-bound testosterone in addition to simply free testosterone. Testosterone is bound very weakly to albumin and is easily attracted to the testosterone receptor when blood perfuses androgen-sensitive tissues. In normal women, the amount of free and weakly bound testosterone rarely exceeds 25% of the total circulating level of testosterone.

The measurement of androstenedione and the androstenedione/DHEAS ratio can also be of use in distinguishing whether the source of the androgen excess is from the ovary or adrenal. In patients with excessive adrenal androgen production, both androstenedione and DHEAS are elevated. In contrast, patients in whom the ovary is the primary source of excess androgen production such as patients with polycystic ovarian disease or patients with an androgen secreting ovarian tumor, androstenedione levels are significantly raised while the level of DHEAS remains relatively normal. Patients with androgen secreting ovarian tumors have elevated testosterone levels as well.

Conclusion

Reproductive disorders in the male and female present with a constellation of symptoms that usually involve abnormal hormone secretion. The site of the disorder is sometimes difficult to identify and thus appropriate laboratory investigation of the patient can help pinpoint the cause of the problem and lead to appropriate therapy. Infertility is one of the major reasons why patients seek medical help with an endocrine problem. However, there are a number of other endocrine disorders that can fulminate if left unrecognized and lead to major metabolic disturbances. Reproductive endocrinology is a discipline that utilizes the laboratory heavily in sorting out a reproductive disorder. Testing of the hypothalamic-pituitary-gonadal axis with provocative stimulation and suppression tests is paramount in many cases to establishing the differential diagnosis. The laboratories ability to produce timely and accurate hormone tests facilitates the diagnosis and treatment of endocrine reproductive disorders.

Table 3. Reference Values for Reproductive Hormones

	FSH (mIu/ml)	LH (mIu/ml)	TESTOSTERONE (ng/dl)	FREE T (ng/dl)	ESTRADIOL (pg/ml)	ESTRONE (pg/ml)
Male	< 20	< 25	250 - 900	110 - 360	15 - 40	45 - 60
Female						
Follicular	< 17	< 20	20 - 80	1 - 15	10 - 100	40 - 210
Luteal	< 12	< 25	—		190 - 340	58 - 200
Menopausal	> 40	> 40	—	10 - 40	24 - 78	

	URINE FSH (mIu/hr)	URINE LH (mIu/hr)	URINE E2 (ug/24 hr)	URINE E1 (ug/24 hr)
Male				
0 - 11 y	10 - 160	10 - 100	—	—
11 - 19	20 - 1310	20 - 1800	—	—
> 20 y	190 - 1700	550 - 2500	—	—
Female				
0 - 11 y	10 - 160	10 - 100	—	—
11 - 19	20 - 1310	20 - 1800	—	—
20 - 49	120 - 1490	190 - 3350	4.0 - 9.0	6.0 - 12
> 50 y	> 1700	> 1000	0.3 - 1.5	1.3 - 6.0

	PROGESTERONE (ng/ml)	17-OH PROGESTERONE (ng/ml)	DHEA-S (ng/ml)	ANDROSTENEDIONE (ng/ml)
Male	0.1 - 0.3	0.3 - 2.1	1,500 - 4,500	0.5 - 2.0
Female				
Follicular	0.2 - 0.9	0.1 - 0.8	1,000 - 3,500	0.4 - 2.4
Luteal	3.0 - 36	0.3 - 2.9	—	—
Menopausal	0.1 - 0.6	0.1 - 0.9	0.5 - 1.3	—

References

1. Carr, B. Disorders of the ovary and female reproductive tract. In. Williams, Textbook of Endocrinology, 8th edition, eds. JD Wilson and DW Foster. WB Saunders, Philadelphia 1992:733-799
2. Griffin, JE and Wilson, JD. Disorders of the testes and the male reproductive tract. In. Williams, Textbook of Endocrinology, 8th edition, eds. JD Wilson and DW Foster. WB Saunders, Philadelphia 1992:799-853.
3. Marshall, JC. Hormonal Regulation of the menstrual cycle and mechanisms of anovulation. In. Endocrinology, 3rd edition, ed. DeGroot, LO. WB Saunders, Philadelphia, 1995:2046-2058
4. Winter, SJ. Clinical disorders of the testis. In Endocrinology, 3rd edition, ed. DeGroot, LO. WB Saunders, Philadelphia, 1995:2377-2403
5. Santner SJ, Santen RJ, Kulin HE and Demers LM: A model for validation of radio-immunoassay kit reagents: Measurement of follitropin and lutropin in blood and urine. Clin Chem 27(11): 1892-1895, 1981
6. Kulin HM, Samojlik E, Demers LM and Santner SO: Response of the prepubertal ovary to acute chorionic gonadotropin administration: Absence of modulation by growth hormone. J Clin Endocrinol Metab 60: 208-211, 1985
7. Lookingbill DP, Horton R, Demers LM, Eagan N, Marks J Jr and Santen RJ: Tissue production of androgens in women with acne. J Am Acad Dermatol 12(3): 481-487, 1985
8. Veldhuis JD, Evans WS, Demers LM, Thorner MO, Wakat D and Rogol AD: Neuroendocrine regulation of gonadotropin secretion in women distance runners. J Clin Endocrinol Metab 61: 557-563, 1985
9. Wild RA, Buchanan JR, Myers C, and Demers LM: Declining adrenal androgens: An association with bone loss in aging women. Proceedings of Society of Experimental Biology Medicine 186: 335-360, 1987
10. Lloyd T, Myers C, Buchanan JR, and Demers LM: Collegiate women athletes with irregular menses during adolescence have decreased bone density. Ob Gyn Vol 72, No. 4, pp 639-642, 1988

11. Baker E. and Demers LM: Menstrual status in female athletes: Correlation with reproductive hormones and bone density. Obstet. Gynec. Vol 72, No. 5, pp 683-687, 1988

12. Buchanan JR, Hospodar P, Myers C, Leuenberger P, and Demers LM: Effect of excess endogenous androgens on bone density in young women. J. Clin Endo Metab. Vol 67, No 5, pp 986-991, 1988

13. Kulin HE, Frontera MA, Demers LM, Lloyd TA, and Bartholomew MJ: The onset of sperm production in pubertal boys: Relation to gonadotropin excretion. Amer J. Disease Children, Vol 143 pp 190-193, 1989

14. Pardridge WM and Demers LM: Bioavailable testosterone in salivary glands. Clin. Chem., 37(2):139-40, 1991

15. Wild RA, Demers LM, Applebaum-Bowden D, and Lenker R: Hirsutism: metabolic effects of two commonly used oral contraceptives and spironolactone. Contraception 44(2):113-24, 1991

16. Brackett LE, Demers LM, Mamourian AC, Ellenberger C, and Santen RJ: Moebius syndrome in association with hypogonadotropic hypogonadism. J. Endocrinol. Invest. 14(7):599-607, 1991

17. DeSouza M J, Luciano AA, Arce JC, Demers LM, Loucks AB: Clinical tests explain blunted cortisol responsiveness but not mild hypercortisolism in amenorrheic runners. J Appl. Physiol 76(3):1302-1309, 1994

18. Kulin H, Demers L, Chinchilli V, Martel J, Stevens L: Usefulness of sequential urine FSH and LH measurements in the diagnosis of adolescent-aged hypogonadotropism. J Clin Endo & Metab. 78(5):1208-1212, 1994

19. Kulin HE, Finkelstein JW, D'Arcangelo MR, Susman EJ, Chinchilli V, Kunselman S, Schwab J, Demers LM, Lookingbill G: Diversity of pubertal testosterone changes in boys with constitutional delay in growth and/or adolescence. J Clin Endo & Metab. 10, 395-400, 1997.

5
Disorders of Mineral Metabolism & Metabolic Bone Disease

MICHAEL KLEEREKOPER, MD & GARY W. EDELSON, MD

Introduction

Metabolic bone disease is a general term which encompasses a broad range of disorders affecting bone metabolism and/or microarchitecture. The most commonly encountered metabolic bone diseases include osteoporosis, Paget's disease, primary hyperparathyroidism, and hyperparathyroidism secondary to renal osteodystrophy, rickets, or osteomalacia. Generally speaking, metabolic bone disease results from disturbances in 1) calcium and/or phosphorus homeostasis or 2) the organic matrix of bone which is comprised of collagen and, to a lesser degree, noncollagenous protein.

Normal bone physiology involves two major cell types, the osteoclasts and the osteoblasts. The osteoclasts are responsible for bone resorption and the osteoblasts are responsible for bone formation. Together they orchestrate bone remodeling. Activation of bone remodeling begins with recruitment of osteoclasts which in turn signal the recruitment of osteoblasts. This relationship is referred to as coupling. Uncoupling of osteoclastic and osteoblastic activity can lead to metabolic bone disease. The bone remodeling process is both under paracrine control and systemic hormonal endocrine control. Few biochemical reactions or physiologic mechanisms can take place properly without an adequate supply of free or ionized calcium intracellularly. In order to ensure that this supply is always adequate, a complex homeostatic system has evolved to ensure that the extracellular (circulating) level of ionized calcium is maintained essentially constant within a very narrow range. The major systemic hormones involved in bone metabolism are parathyroid hormone(PTH) and vitamin D.

Parathyroid hormone is a single-chain, 84-amino acid polypeptide secreted by the parathyroid glands in response to a fall in serum ionized calcium. As depicted in Figure 1, it has three major effects, two of which are direct and one of which is indirect. The direct effects of PTH are to stimulate osteoclastic cellular activity, thereby increasing the rate of bone resorption and increasing serum calcium and phosphate, and the other is to increase calcium reabsorption in the proximal renal tubules which also increases serum calcium. Both of these actions serve to increase the concentration of ionic calcium in the serum and extracellular fluid. PTH also causes phosphaturia thereby lowering serum phosphate concentrations. The indirect effect of parathyroid hormone is that it promotes the pro-

FIGURE 1. THE HORMONAL CONTROL OF SERUM CALCIUM IS DEPICTED.

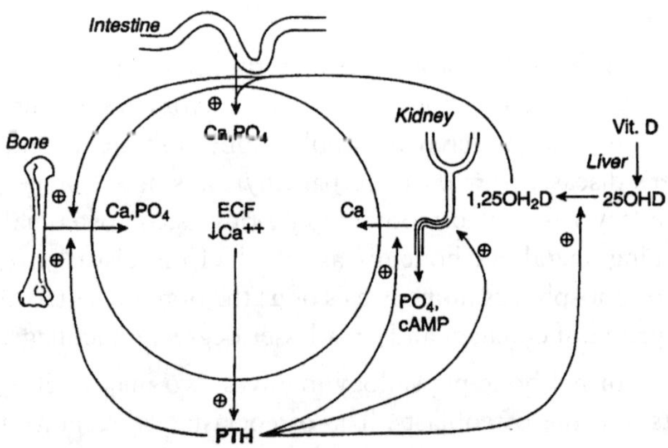

ECF = extracellular fluid; Ca = calcium; PO4 = phosphate; cAMP = cyclic adenosine monophosphate; PTH = parathyroid hormone; 25OHD = calcidiol; and 1,25 OH2D = calcitriol

From Edelson GW, Kleerekoper MD. Hypercalcemic Crisis. Page 81. Endocrine Emergencies. Medical Clinics of North America Vol 79, Number 1, January 1995.

duction of calcitriol (1,25-dihydroxyvitamin D) in the kidneys via the activation of α1-hydroxylase. Calcitriol in turn promotes calcium and phosphate absorption from the small intestine. It is also known that calcitriol is responsible for many other activities including effects on osteoclastic bone resorption, monocyte and myelocyte maturation and differentiation, insulin secretion and osteocalcin production, to name a few. Osteocalcin, also known as bone glutamic acid (GLA) containing protein, is the most abundant noncollagenous matrix protein of bone whose physiological significance is unknown. It serves as a very specific marker of osteoblastic activity as it is almost exclusively produced by osteoblasts. Calcitriol also has a direct inhibitory effect via negative feedback on parathyroid tissue and parathyroid hormone secretion. The net effect of PTH in patients with normal renal function is to raise serum calcium and lower serum inorganic phosphate. Total body phosphate is ultimately controlled by the rate of renal phosphate excretion and by gastrointestinal absorption with at least 70% of dietary phosphate being absorbed.

The hormone calcitonin, synthesized and secreted by the parafollicular C-cells of the thyroid gland, is often included in discussions of the calciotropic hormones. However, since the precise physiologic role of calcitonin in humans is unknown, it will not be further discussed in this chapter other than to mention that it serves as a tumor marker for medullary thyroid carcinoma.

In addition to hormonal control of the calcium concentration, there is physical-chemical control. The physical-chemical control of serum calcium involves the binding of calcium to protein, predominantly albumin, and to a lesser extent globulins, and the influences of acid base balance on this protein binding of calcium. Ninety-eight to 99% of body stores of calcium are in the skeleton and it is this organ that is asked to pay the price needed to keep the extracellular calcium level constant when the homeostatic systems break down. In other circumstances, there are primary abnormalities in bone metabolism which result in secondary changes in the homeostatic control of extracellular calcium.

Derangements of the hormonal system which regulates serum calcium levels can result in either hyper or hypocalcemia. Hypercalcemia can broadly be classified as PTH and non-PTH mediated disease with primary hyperparathyroidism being by far the most common cause (Table 1). Primary hyperparathyroidism is caused by a single adenoma in 80% of cases, by four gland hyperplasia in nearly 20% of cases, and by parathyroid carcinoma in fewer than 1% of cases. Other possible etiologies

TABLE 1. DIFFERENTIAL DIAGNOSIS OF HYPERCALCEMIA

PARATHYROID MEDIATED
Primary hyperparathyroidism
adenoma
hyperplasia
carcinoma
"Tertiary" hyperparathyroidism
complicating longstanding secondary hyperparathyroidism
post-renal transplant
long-term phosphate therapy for hypophosphatemic rickets

NON-PARATHYROID MEDIATED
Malignant disease
Solid tissue malignancy with or without bone metastases (PTHrP)
Widespread osteolytic metastases (not PTHrP mediated)
Hematologic malignancy (TNF, OAF)
Lymphoma (?calcitriol)
Endocrine disease
Addison's disease
Hypo- or hyperthyroidism
Williams syndrome
Medications
Vitamin D excess
Vitamin A excess
Thiazide diuretics (may be PTH mediated)
Lithium (may be PTH mediated)
Milk-alkali syndrome
Granulomatous disease
Miscellaneous
Familial hypocalciuric hypercalcemia (FHH)
Immobilization
children
adolescents
Paget's disease of bone
Recovery from acute renal failure of rhabdomyolysis

for PTH mediated hypercalcemia include familial hypocalciuric hypercalcemia (FHH), lithium and thiazide diuretic induced hypercalcemia, and tertiary hyperparathyroidism. Non-PTH medicated hypercalcemia is most commonly due to malignancy mediated through various humoral mechanisms such as parathyroid related peptide (PTHrP), 1, 25-dihydroxyvitamin

D, and osteoclast activating factor (OAF). Less frequently, malignancy through local osteolysis can cause hypercalcemia when there is fairly extensive metastatic disease. Granulomatous diseases (via endogenous vitamin D intoxication), endocrine disorders (such as thyrotoxicosis and pheochromocytoma), vitamin D intoxication and immobilization can all cause hypercalcemia.

In general terms, hypocalcemia is due either to PTH or vitamin D deficiency or resistance (Table 2). Deficiency of PTH can be induced surgically or by neck irradiation, it may be due to congenital absence of parathyroid tissue, caused by infiltrative or autoimmune (idiopathic) disease, or metabolically, by hypomagnesemia. Hypomagnesemia, in addition, results in a degree of PTH resistance so intact PTH levels may be normal or high. Vitamin D deficiency can be caused by substrate deficiency in any step along the pathway of vitamin D metabolism or by effects on any of the enzymes involved in the metabolic steps in the production of 1,25-dihydroxyvitamin D. The PTH resistance syndromes, also referred to as pseudohypoparathyroidism, are characterized by hypocalcemia and hyperphosphatemia in the face of an elevated PTH level. Even less frequently encountered is the autosomal recessively inherited syndrome of resistance to 1,25-dihydroxyvitamin D that is the cause of vitamin D rickets.

Biochemical Testing

General Considerations

The pertinent biochemical tests employed in the diagnosis and evaluation of patients for metabolic bone disease include assessments of serum and urine calcium, phosphate, parathyroid hormone levels, vitamin D metabolite levels, and the measurement of markers which provide insight into the relative degree of activity of the osteoclasts and osteoblasts. Available markers include end products of enzymatic activity specific for osteoblasts or osteoclasts and the metabolites of the bone collagen organic matrix as listed in Table 3. The synthesis and secretion of parathyroid hormone and calcitriol are so intimately linked to the control of serum calcium and inorganic phosphate (and of course skeletal metabolism), that their measurement should never be obtained in the absence of concurrent data concerning serum calcium and inorganic phosphate. This close relationship obviates the need for stimulation or suppression tests commonly employed in other endocrinologic evaluations. Additionally, since calcitriol is synthesized and secreted by the kidney and has such a dominant role in par-

TABLE 2. DIFFERENTIAL DIAGNOSIS OF HYPOCALCEMIA

PARATHYROID HORMONE DEFICIENCY

associated with hyperphosphatemia and normal alkaline phosphatase

- Congenital
  - isolated
  - Di George syndrome
- Neonatal (transient)
- Acquired
  - idiopathic
  - autoimmune
  - post-surgical
  - infiltrative diseases
    - metastases
    - hemosiderosis/hemochromatosis
  - hypomagnesemia

PARATHYROID HORMONE EXCESS

associated with hyperphosphatemia ± elevated alkaline phosphatase

- Parathyroid hormone resistance
  - Pseudohypoparathyroidism
    - type I
    - type IIa
    - type IIb
  - Chronic renal failure (late)
  - Drug-induced
    - phosphate infusion
    - phosphate enema

associated with hypophosphatemia and elevated alkaline phosphatase

- Calcediol deficiency
  - malnutrition
  - malabsorption
  - very limited sunlight exposure
  - chronic liver disease
- Calcitriol deficiency
  - vitamin D dependent rickets
- Phosphate
  - hypophosphatemic rickets (or "vitamin D resistant rickets")
  - Fanconi syndrome
- Drug-induced
  - Calcitonin
  - Bisphosphonates
  - Cisplatinum
- Miscellaneous (PTH status not fully determined)
  - Massive transfusion with citrated blood
  - Acute pancreatitis

TABLE 3. BIOCHEMICAL MARKERS OF BONE TURNOVER

FORMATION (OSTEOBLASTIC)	RESORPTION (OSTEOCLASTIC)
Serum osteocalcin (bone GLA protein)	Urinary calcium excretion
Total and bone-specific alkaline phosphatase	Urinary hydroxypoline
Serum procollagen I extension peptides (PICP)	Urinary pyridinoline and deoxy-pyridinoline (collagen crosslinks)
	Urinary hydroxylysine glycosides
	Urinary pyridinoline crosslinked amino-telopeptides (NTX)
	Serum pyridinoline crosslinked carboxy-telopeptides (ICTP)
	Plasma tartrate-resistant acid phosphatase (TRAP)

athyroid hormone synthesis and secretion, it is also essential to have concomitant data concerning glomerular filtration rate. A measurement of serum creatinine generally suffices for this assessment of renal function.

Measurement of Calcium in Serum and Urine

The reference interval for serum calcium in normal adults is 8.8 to 10.2 mg/dL with very slight fluctuation from one laboratory to the next depending upon the subjects used to determine the reference interval and the method of measurement of calcium. While the 95% confidence interval for calcium encompasses 1.4 mg/dL, day-to-day, week-to-week and month-to-month fluctuations in individual subjects should not exceed ±0.5 mg/dL or less. Of the total serum calcium concentration, approximately 50% is in the free or ionized form, 45% is protein bound, and 5% is chelated or complexed. Approximately 80-90% of the calcium that is bound to protein is bound to albumin and 10-20% is bound to globulin. Alterations in serum proteins affect the portion of total serum calcium that is protein bound, always with the emphasis being the constancy of the serum ionized calcium concentration. Several nomograms and complex formulae are available to "normalize" the total serum calcium for protein binding with the most widely used being: corrected total calcium concentration(mg/dL) = measured total calcium concentration(mg/dL) + 0.8 x [4.0 - serum albumin concentration(gm/dL)]. In the modern clinical chemistry laboratory, even the most complex of formulae can be incorporated into the computer programs of automated biochemical analyzers to calculate the most precise estimate of ionized and protein bound calcium. This is particularly relevant in circumstances where there are extreme abnormalities in serum proteins, particularly severe hypoalbuminemia or hyperglobulinemia.

The only physiologically relevant calcium concentration is that of the free or ionized component. It would seem most logical to measure ionized calcium directly via sensitive ion specific electrodes that would obviate the need for protein binding corrections. This technology has been available for more than two decades. However, there are several practical reasons that limit its use. Most importantly the specimen must be collected and analyzed anaerobically. While all available ionized calcium electrodes can and do normalize the result for a blood pH of 7.4, this is still only meaningful if the specimen is analyzed anaerobically. This requirement makes it impractical to put ionized calcium "on line" with other automated profiles. Either a separate specimen for ionized calcium measurement should be specifically collected from the patient or the aliquot for ionized calcium should be removed by a needle and syringe before the seal on the vaccutainer is broken. In most busy clinical chemistry laboratories, it is adequate to measure total calcium and albumin (or total protein) and calculate corrected calcium by the formulae: Corrected calcium = measured calcium – 0.8 (albumin – 4.5) / Corrected calcium = measured calcium – 0.5 (protein – 7.5).

Measurement of calcium in the urine is a simple analytic procedure, but the interpretation of the result requires some discussion. Reference intervals for urine calcium are not as well established as those for serum calcium, but a value of 4 mg/kg body weight per day is generally regarded as the upper limit of normal. Whenever a 24 hour urine collection is obtained for measurement of calcium, it is essential that both excretion of creatinine and sodium be included in the analysis. Creatinine should be an integral part of any 24 hour urine measurement as an assessment of the adequacy of collection. Under most circumstances, the renal tubules handle calcium and sodium together such that any tendency towards natriuresis also produces calciuresis. This is of particular concern in patients with hypercalciuria which, if accompanied by hypernatriuria, may simply reflect increased dietary sodium intake or diuretic natriuresis from loop of Henle blockers. Of the diuretics in common use, furosemide promotes hypercalciuria while thiazide diuretics limit the renal excretion of calcium.

Assays for Calciotropic Hormones

Parathyroid Hormone

Parathyroid hormone (PTH) is an 84 amino acid single chain polypeptide and is the hormone par excellence of which structure/function relationships influence the choice and development of immunoassays. The biologic action of PTH resides in the first 34 amino acids at the amino terminus, but this peptide has such a short half-life that assays for the amino terminal fragment are of limited clinical utility. The major circulating PTH fragment is the carboxyterminal (C-terminal) fragment, but clearance of this fragment is so influenced by the glomerular filtration rate that use of immunoassays directed against the carboxyterminal portion of the PTH molecule have fallen into disfavor. Renal failure, even in the absence of hyperparathyroidism, will elevate C-terminal PTH. In the last decade, highly sensitive and specific sandwich immunoradiometric (IRMA) and immunochemiluminescent (ICMA) assays have been developed for measurement of the intact 1 to 84 amino acid sequence of PTH. Assays for intact PTH are not significantly influenced by renal function and as such have been demonstrated to clearly reflect PTH secretion. It is appropriate to state categorically that at the present time there is little if any indication for continued use of any assay for PTH other than the intact PTH assay. A recent report suggests that intact PTH or epitopes measured by the IRMA or ICMA for intact PTH may accumulate in patients with renal failure. This has not yet been confirmed. Assays for intact PTH are readily available through most large commercial clinical chemistry laboratories and kits for in-house performance of assays are also readily available.

Vitamin D Metabolites

Calcidiol (25-hydroxyvitamin D) is a metabolite of vitamin D whose measure provides an assessment of vitamin D stores. This is not a particularly potent hormone binding to the nuclear vitamin D receptor with only 1×10^{-3} the affinity with which calcitriol (1,25 dihydroxyvitamin D) binds to the same receptor. However, the circulating concentration of calcidiol measured in ng/ml is one thousand fold the circulating concentration of calcitriol measured in pg/ml. Calcidiol is synthesized in the liver from the precursor pro-vitamin D and its metabolism can be affected by liver dysfunction and by drugs that influence the cytochrome P450 oxidase system. Because calcidiol is in great excess relative to the formation of calcitriol, in the absence of decreased hepatic bile secretion, liver dysfunction doesn't usually significantly disturb vitamin D metabolism. Calcidiol is measured by radioimmunoassay (RIA). As with PTH, commercial assays and kits for 25- hydroxyvitamin D are readily available. An RIA method for measurement of 1,25 dihydroxyvitamin D has recently been developed and has supplanted the older competitive protein binding assays that relied heavily on HPLC. Commercial assays and kits are also readily available.

Assays for markers of bone remodeling

Currently available markers of bone formation include alkaline phosphatase, osteocalcin, and procollagen type I extension peptides. Bone specific alkaline phosphatase (BSAP) is a specific gene product of the osteoblasts. The precise physiologic function of the bone specific alkaline phosphatase is unknown. Nevertheless, it is a utilitarian marker of osteoblast function. Unfortunately, due to the fact that bone specific alkaline phosphatase cross reacts with the liver isoenzymes of alkaline phosphatase, it is not a very specific marker of bone formation. Certainly, however, the bone specific alkaline phosphatase is much more sensitive than the total alkaline phosphatase and significantly higher levels have been demonstrated in postmenopausal women and in patients with Paget's disease of bone. Levels of this osteoblast marker also are useful in assessing the efficacy of various therapies employed in Paget's disease as well as in the treatment and prevention of osteoporosis.

Osteocalcin (bone GLA protein) is another specific gene product of the osteoblasts. It is the most abundant noncollagenous protein found in bone. It is directly synthesized and secreted by the osteoblasts and then incorporated into the bone matrix. Unfortunately, osteocalcin levels increase during bone resorption as well as bone formation which limits its specificity as a marker of bone formation. It is, therefore, better thought of as a marker of bone turnover rather than specifically bone formation. A lesser problem with osteocalcin is the fact that it is cleared by the kidneys and therefore levels in patients with impaired renal function tend to be higher. Interestingly, 1,25-dihydroxyvitamin D promotes the synthesis of osteocalcin.

Type I collagen makes up more than 90% of the organic matrix of bone. It is synthesized by the osteoblast as a procollagen molecule, but prior to insertion into the extracellular matrix amino-terminal and carboxy-terminal propeptide extensions are proteolytically cleaved. Both the carboxy-terminal propeptide of Type I procollagen and the amino-terminal propeptide of Type I collagen are released into the circulation and are separately measurable. Results of clinical studies with assays employing a radioimmunoassay kit and an ELISA method for measurement of these peptides have not been encouraging in that their results were discordant and inferior to OCN and BSAP for assessing changes in bone formation; however, ongoing research is necessary before any conclusions can be reached.

As can be seen in Table 3, the number of assays available for assessing bone resorption is greater than the number available for bone formation. The major constituents released from the skeleton through bone resorption are calcium and Type I collagen. These products are ultimately cleared by the kidney and, therefore, urinary studies often prove most useful for their measurement. Urinary calcium excretion during a 24 hour period reflects both the net result of dietary calcium absorption as well as skeletal loss of calcium. It has been shown, however, that with at least 12 hours of fasting, the contribution from calcium absorption diminishes and hence fasting urinary calcium excretion much more accurately reflects skeletal loss than does a total 24 hour urine excretion calculation. An increased level in the fasting calcium to creatinine ratio above 0.15 mg/mg creatinine is likely to be associated with increased bone turnover, but this is not a very specific assessment. Probably most importantly, measurement of urinary calcium excretion is the least expensive and the most readily available of all the markers of bone resorption. Tartrate resistant acid phosphatase is an enzyme released from osteoclasts into the circulation. It becomes unstable when frozen and it lacks specificity so it is not widely touted as a clinically useful marker of bone resorption. Hydroxyproline, on the other hand, being the predominant amino acid component of Type I collagen is a very useful assay for assessing bone resorption. With increased bone resorption, urinary hydroxyproline excretion increases. Because hydroxyproline is also a major constituent of other types of collagen, as well as a component of the complement pathway, a significant proportion in the urine comes from these sources. This, in addition to the fact that its measurement is affected by dietary protein intake, gives it fairly limited specificity. It has been shown, however, that after a twelve hour or greater fast, the dietary collagen effects can be sufficiently eliminated.

More recently, assays for the collagen crosslinking amino acids that are excreted in the urine have been developed and have become widely used both in research and clinical settings. Pyridinoline, a nonreducible, trivalent crosslink that stabilizes Type I collagen chains, is released during the degradation of collagen fibrils, and is excreted in the urine. When lysine is incorporated into the collagen crosslink, an analog of pyridinoline, deoxypyridinoline, is formed. Pyridinoline is present in the skeleton more abundantly than is deoxypyridinoline, but deoxypyridinoline is a more specific marker of bone resorption because pyridinoline is also a component of Type II collagen, cartilage, and other connective tissues. Compared to urinary calcium or hydroxyproline assays, however, both of these assays are more specific for bone resorption. Even more recently, several antibody based assays for crosslinking peptides have been developed. These techniques can identify either of the free crosslinking amino acids (pyridinoline and deoxypyridinoline). There is another immunoassay that detects the amino-terminal domain and is referred to as the N-telopeptide of Type I collagen (NTX) assay and that which detects the carboxy-terminal region crosslink is known as the carboxy-terminal telopeptide of Type I collagen (ICTP). Oftentimes the assay employed for measuring ICTP is referred to as the urinary crosslaps assay which actually recognizes a short sequence of amino acids within the entire ICTP chain. Although these assays are not affected greatly by diurnal variation, there still is significant intraindividual variation. Thus, these newer urinary and serum markers for measuring collagen crosslinks and telopeptides are more sensitive markers of bone turnover than the older serum and urinary markers, but they have practical limitations which prohibit their widespread clinical use.

Finally, the amino acid hydroxylysine, which is involved in collagen metabolism, can be measured as the more specific bone component known as galactosyl hydroxylysine. However, the performance of this assay is quite cumbersome and therefore is of limited use and availability.

Pathophysiology

General Considerations

There are literally hundreds of publications that document significant correlations between the various aforementioned biochemical markers and metabolic bone disease. In the clinical setting of metabolic bone disease, the measurement of calcitrophic hormones is much more important and useful than are the measurements of the markers of bone remodeling. Table 4 summarizes the biochemical findings in metabolic bone disease.

Primary Hyperparathyroidism

This primary disorder of parathyroid hormone secretion results from clonal growth of parathyroid cells that are still under the control of the prevailing serum ionized calcium concentration, but at a higher set point. The biochemical hallmark of primary hyperparathyroidism is persistent hypercalcemia. In patients with primary hyperparathyroidism, the mean serum calcium concentration is almost invariably above the reference interval for normals, but occasionally in patients with mild disease, individual values for serum calcium may be within the normal reference interval albeit towards the upper range of normal. Serum intact PTH is elevated above the normal reference interval in 80% or more of patients with primary hyperparathyroidism depending on the series quoted. This means that in up to 20% of patients, the serum intact PTH may be within the normal reference interval. However, with very few exceptions, intact PTH is in the top half of the normal reference interval. Most importantly, in nonparathyroid hypercalcemia, serum intact PTH is almost always suppressed with the measured level below the lower limit of the reference interval. PTH depresses the tubular maximum for phosphate reabsorption and therefore serum inorganic phosphate is generally, but not always, low in this disease. The hypercalcemia of primary hyperparathyroidism increases the filtered load of calcium tending to increase urinary calcium excretion. At the same time, the excess parathyroid hormone synthesis and secretion enhances renal tubular absorption of calcium tending to lower the urinary excretion of calcium. Thus, the net urinary calcium excretion in primary hyperparathyroidism may be normal, or as is more common, elevated. This is in contrast to nonparathyroid hypercalcemia where urinary calcium excretion is invariably elevated. PTH has direct stimulatory action on osteoclasts and osteoblasts and thus the biochemical markers of bone remodeling (as discussed in the previous section) are generally elevated in primary hyperparathyroidism. Because parathyroid hormone increases renal alpha 1-hydroxylase activity, 1,25-dihydroxyvitamin D levels tend to be elevated, but 25-hydroxyvitamin D levels are normal.

In the presence of normal renal function, there are only two hypercalcemic conditions that are not associated with hypercalciuria. The most common cause is primary hyperparathyroidism. Infrequently, a patient with familial (benign) hypocalciuric hypercalcemia (FHH) will be encountered who manifests hypercalcemia, low normal PTH, and usually very low urine calcium (e.g., <50 mg/24 hours). This disorder results from an abnormality in the recently discovered calcium-sensing receptor gene. Discovery of FHH in a hypercalcemic proband should lead to measurement of serum calcium in family members. Unlike primary hyperparathyroidism, FHH is not associated with nephrocalcinosis or the development of renal failure and the hypercalcemia is not corrected by parathyroidectomy. For that reason, surgery is contraindicated.

Secondary Hyperparathyroidism

There are diverse etiologies for a secondary compensatory increase in parathyroid hormone secretion. In all of these conditions, serum intact PTH is elevated above the reference interval in response to a decline in ionized calcium resulting from decreased calcium absorption. Because of the compensatory rise in PTH, calcium is normal (or low), but is never elevated in secondary hyperparathyroidism. The etiology of decreased calcium absorption is a deficiency in serum calcidiol and/or calcitriol. Calcidiol deficiency generally complicates intestinal disease (malabsorption, malnutrition, or short bowel syndrome) when vitamin D is malabsorbed. Deficiency of calcidiol impairs calcium absorption eliciting an increase in PTH which in turn acts as a stimulus to the renal alpha-1-hydroxylase enzyme increasing production of calcitriol. Increased calcitriol production improves calcium absorption. In early stages of secondary hyperparathyroidism, even though serum calcidiol levels are low, the serum calcium will be normal, but the serum PTH will be elevated and the major biochemical abnormality will be an increase in serum alkaline phosphatase reflecting the stimulatory effect of PTH on osteoblast function. Urinary calcium excretion will be low. As the disease progresses, there is further reduction in circulating calcidiol levels, but the serum calcium remains normal until such time as calcidiol levels have fallen sufficiently to lower serum calcitriol levels. In other words, it is only when calcitriol levels are low that serum calcium falls below normal. This is clearly a late stage of the disease. The primary mechanism whereby liver disease produces secondary hyperparathyroidism is decreased bile acid excretion and vitamin D malabsorption ensues.

The second and certainly most common cause of secondary hyperparathyroidism is chronic renal failure. As shown in Figure 2 there is progressive decline in the alpha-1-hydroxylase enzyme activity, a subsequent decline in calcitriol levels, and a progressive stimulation of PTH in an attempt to maintain normal calcitriol levels necessary for intestinal calcium absorption. Since calcitriol is essential for proper absorption of calcium in the gastrointestinal tract, serum calcium tends to be low earlier in this form of secondary hyperparathyroidism than in hyperparathyroidism secondary to calcidiol deficiency. Initially, when creatinine clearance is above 30 to 35 ml/min, the effect of parathyroid hormone on the tubular maximum (Tm) for phosphate is still observed and there will be mild hypophosphatemia. However, as renal function declines further, there is phosphate retention which results in hyperphosphatemia. This aggravates the hypocalcemia via in vivo precipitation of calcium-phophate complexes (ectopic calcification) and suppresses alpha-1-hydroxylase enzyme activity further lowering serum calcitriol and aggravating the secondary hyperparathyroidism. Because of secondary hyperparathyroidism, bone remodeling rates are increased and as such the markers of both bone resorption and formation generally are elevated.

The treatment of choice in calcidiol deficiency is clearly calcidiol while the treatment of choice for calcitriol deficiency is equally clearly calcitriol. The bone disease resulting from calcidiol deficiency in adults is osteomalacia with accompanying secondary hyperparathyroidism whereas children develop rickets. Because of the slowly evolving nature of this disease, there is generally a marked increase in the amount of nonmineralized bone matrix. Early in the course of therapy, this

FIGURE 2. CHRONIC RENAL FAILURE

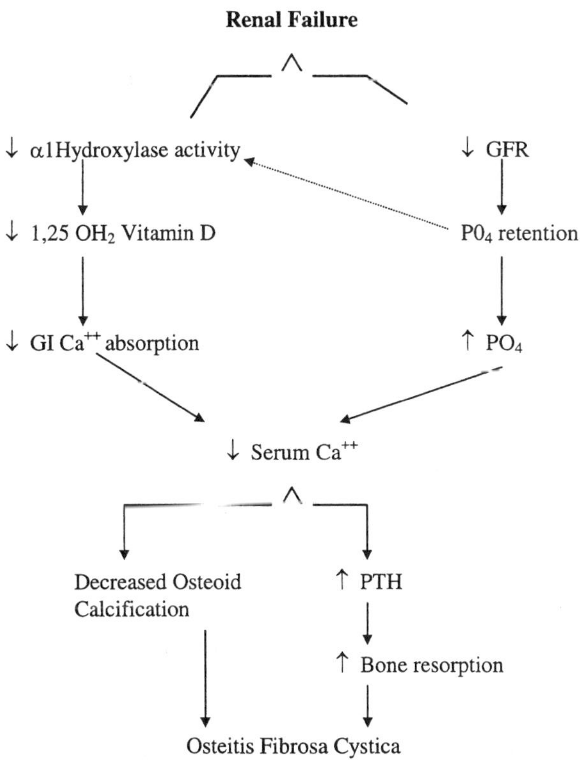

nonmineralized matrix becomes increasingly mineralized, but during this process, it serves as a sump for calcium and there will be an initial fall in serum calcium and inorganic phosphate as the osteoid becomes progressively more mineralized. This in turn will be accompanied by a further increase in the alkaline phosphatase (the so called "phosphatase flare") reflecting further stimulation of osteoblast function as the bone is healing. The restoration of normal serum calcium and normal urinary calcium will not occur until the skeleton is more fully mineralized. This is usually preceded by a reversal of the alkaline phosphatase flare as bone healing continues.

Hypophosphatemic states can also cause rickets or osteomalacia of which there are various genetic and acquired etiologies. Hyperphosphaturia is the classic finding in these conditions. There are two types of vitamin D dependent rickets or osteomalacia. The first type results from a failure, deficiency, or abnormality of the renal alpha-1-hydroxylase enzyme resulting in a deficiency of calcitriol. In this disorder, the calcidiol levels tend to be normal and as expected, the calcitriol levels are clearly low. In the second type of vitamin D dependent rickets or osteomalacia, there is end organ resistance to the action of calcitriol. In this condition, both the calcidiol and calcitriol levels are normal or high. Renal tubular acidosis, long term anticonvulsant use (toxic hepatic hydroxylation), liver disease (hepatic rickets), Fanconi syndrome, and bone or soft tissue tumors are other less common causes of rickets and osteomalacia. In pediatric practice in the United States, the most common cause of rickets is vitamin D resistant rickets caused by an X-linked dominant renal tubular failure to conserve phosphate (i.e. familial hypophosphatemic rickets). Nutritional rickets is rare in the U.S.

Paget's Disease

Paget's disease results from excessive osteoclastic bone resorption followed by an exuberant increase in osteoblastic activity. There is such avid bone remodeling occurring that the new bone which is formed is haphazard in its architecture, expanded, and structurally incompetent. It is a fairly common disease with a slight male predominanace occuring especially in those of European and North American descent who are over the age of 55. It is thought to be caused by a paramyxovirus infection of the osteoclasts. Paget's disease may affect a single bone in which case it is referred to as monostotic disease or multiple bones which is referred to as polyostotic disease. The most common presentation of disease is that of an asymptomatic patient who is detected with an elevated serum alkaline phosphatase level on routine biochemical screening. The remainder of the metabolic bone disease laboratory parameters are normal. The most common symptomatic presentation is bone pain. Complications from Paget's disease are quite common and include pathologic as well as nonpathologic fractures, nerve entrapment syndromes, osteoarthritis of joints adjacent to pagetic bone, conductive hearing loss, and rarely, high output congestive heart failure due to extreme hypervascularity of involved bone and osteosarcoma.

Because there is such avid osteoclastic bone resorption and osteoblastic bone formation in Paget's disease, the biochemical markers of bone remodeling which reflect the levels of bone formation and bone resorption are usually significantly elevated and valuable in the diagnosis as well as in the monitoring of patients with this disease. Although radionuclide bone scanning and plain x-rays are the only accurate means of identifying pagetic lesions in bone, it is the markers of bone remodeling which allow for the evaluation of the degree of disease activity. In general, the more extensive the disease, the higher the levels of bone markers. Traditionally, serum alkaline phosphatase levels and 24 hour urinary hydroxyproline excretion rates have been used for diagnosing and monitoring disease. However, with the advent of more sensitive indicators of bone remodeling, these have become almost outdated. Bone specific alkaline phosphatase (BSAP), of all the available bone formation markers, is the most sensitive. The assays for measuring levels of the collagen crosslinking amino acids, pyridinoline and deoxypyridinoline, or the NTX or ICTP assays, are the best markers for assessing the degree of bone resorption.

In general, the various available treatments of Paget's disease target the osteoclast. Through inhibition of osteoclastic activity, there is a direct reduction in bone resorption and an indirect reduction in bone formation. Injectable salmon and human calcitonin are effective in Paget's disease resulting in thirty to fifty percent reductions in serum alkaline phosphatase and urinary hydroxyproline levels within three to six months of starting treatment. The problem with salmon calcitonin is that it must be given by injection which is usually not readily accepted by patients, its use is complicated by fairly significant and frequent side effects, and almost half of the salmon calcitonin treated patients will develop resistance to treatment over time.

Currently, in the United States, there are five Food and Drug Administration (FDA) approved bisphosphonates for the treatment of Paget's disease. These include etidronate, alendronate, pamidronate, tiludronate and residronate. These agents inhibit osteoclastic bone resorption and secondarily decrease osteoblastic activity and overall bone remodeling. Etidronate is a first generation bisphosphonate which can be administered orally continuously for up to six months. Up to sixty percent of patients will respond with a significant reduction in serum alkaline phosphatase levels. However, the third generation bisphosphonate, alendronate, is much more potent and does not appear to have the potential for causing osteomalacia as does the former. Orally administered alendronate has been shown to significantly decrease both serum alkaline phosphatase and urinary deoxypyridinoline levels in approximately 75% of treated patients. The second generation bisphosphonate, pamidronate, likewise has been shown to significantly reduce markers of bone remodeling in approximately 3/4 of treated patients. Finally, another second generation bisphosphonate, tiludronate, which only recently became available for the treatment of Paget's disease, also causes 50-60% reductions in serum alkaline phosphatase levels. What is true of all the therapeutic agents thus far discussed is that the response to therapy is somewhat dependent on the initial degree of elevation of the bone markers. In other words, those who have higher concentrations of the bone remodeling biochemical markers are likely to be more resistant to therapy and will require repeated or prolonged therapeutic intervention.

Osteoporosis

Osteoporosis results from remodeling imbalances where resorption outstrips formation. During childhood and adolescence, the skeleton is in positive balance (when bone formation exceeds bone resorption). Once peak adult bone mass is achieved during the second to fourth decades of life, the skeleton is in balance for a short period of time, probably less than ten years. Thereafter, there is always negative skeletal balance leading to the universal phenomenon of age-related bone loss. If left unperturbed, eventually we would all become old enough to develop osteoporosis. During age-related bone loss, which is quite slow at <1% of bone mass lost per year, the changes in the rate of remodeling are subtle giving rise to what has been termed "low turnover bone loss". Many skeletal insults activate the remodeling process, widening the imbalance between resorption and formation giving rise to "high turnover bone loss" which exceeds 1% per year, at least for short periods. In high turnover bone loss, the imbalance per unit of remodeling remains constant, but the number of units undergoing remodeling at any one time is increased.

Diseases that activate remodeling and lead to high turnover bone loss include hormone excess (cortisol, parathyroid hormone, thyroxine), hormone deficiency (estrogen, testosterone, and the vitamin D metabolites), immobilization, malignancy (skeletal metastases, multiple myeloma), and some uncommon diseases such as systemic mastocytosis. Many medications also activate remodeling and increase bone turnover and bone loss. These include glucocorticosteroids, thyroxine, anticonvulsants, antimetabolites, and anticoagulants such as heparin.

The biochemical markers of bone remodeling previously discussed cannot accurately assess bone mass. Since low bone mass and increased skeletal fragility are the hallmarks of osteoporosis, these markers cannot be used to establish the diagnosis. However, there is mounting evidence that for any given bone mass, the rate of remodeling is an independent predictor of the likelihood of sustaining a subsequent osteoporotic fragility fracture. Studies in older individuals (age > 75 years) have indeed demonstrated that a low level of the bone resorption marker ICTP can predict fracture risk independent of bone mass. This is important, but still insufficient to permit the use of the markers for diagnostic purposes even in the elderly. The current accepted definition of osteoporosis is that it is *a systemic disease manifested by low bone mass, microarchitectural deterioration of the skeleton, leading to enhanced bone fragility and a subsequent increase in fracture risk*. The basis of this definition is low bone mass which can only be established by direct densitometric assessment of bone mass and certainly not by biochemical assessment.

In general, the rates of remodeling and bone loss are related such that the higher the turnover, the greater the rate of loss. Therefore, the biochemical markers of bone metabolism (see Table 3) can be used in conjunction with bone mass measurement to predict future bone mass, and to ascertain whether bone mass is being lost at a normal or accelerated rate. Thus, in the evaluation and management of patients with osteoporosis and other metabolic bone diseases, the major role for the biochemical markers is to assist physicians in making appropriate decisions about initiating therapy and monitoring the therapeutic response. It has been recently demonstrated that early postmenopausal women with low turnover (lowest quartile) do not lose bone during one year of therapy with calcium alone, nor gain bone with estrogen therapy. In contrast, those in the top quartile of turnover lose bone most rapidly on calcium alone and gain the greatest amount of bone on estrogen. Earlier studies had demonstrated a similar relationship between the rate of bone turnover and the response to therapy with the anti-resorptive drug calcitonin. There is a similar relationship between early biochemical responses and later increases in bone mass with bisphosphonates as well.

Table 4. Biochemical Findings in Metabolic Bone Diseases

CONDITION	SERUM CALCIUM	SERUM PHOSPHORUS	INTACT PTH	24 HR. URINARY CALCIUM	25 OH VIT. D	1,25 OH_2 VIT. D	MARKERS OF BONE TURNOVER
Primary Hyperparathyroidism	↑	↓/low normal	↑/high normal	↑/N	N	↑	↑
Familial Hypocalciuric Hypercalcemia	↑	N	N/↑	↓	N	N	N
Osteoporosis	N	N	N	N	N	N	↑/N/↓
Paget's Disease	N	N	N	N/↑	N	N	↑
Secondary Hyperparathyroidism—							
GI Disease	N/↓	↓	↑	↓	↓	N/↓	↑
Secondary Hyperparathyroidism—							
Renal Failure	↓/N	↑	↑	↓	N	↓	↑
Rickets/Osteomalacia	↓	N/↓	↑	↓	N/↑/↓	↓/N/↑	↑

There remain several technical difficulties with assays for biochemical markers of bone remodeling that limit their clinical utility. Of particular importance is the diurnal variation in the urine based markers of resorption with values peaking in the morning. This requirement for early morning urine samples (first or second void) is problematic for many older women with osteoporosis and also requires a separate visit to the laboratory to deliver the specimen. The urine markers are all normalized for urine creatinine excretion compounding problems with biologic and assay variability. Overall there is a 20-30% variability in these urine based markers of resorption of similar magnitude to the variability of other urine based studies in endocrinology. The serum based markers of bone formation are not subject to the same diurnal variation and their biologic variability is less at 7-12%. Given this, it would seem most logical to rely more heavily on the formation markers, bone specific alkaline phosphatase (BSAP) and osteocalcin (OCN). There are, however, several biologic and technical limitations to this approach. It has been difficult to develop antibodies to BSAP that do not have substantial cross-reactivity (6-16%) with other alkaline phosphatase isoenzymes, particularly the hepatic moiety which differs from BSAP only in post-translational glycosylation. OCN circulates as an intact molecule and in several fragment forms. OCN also undergoes carboxylation and both carboxylated and uncarboxylated forms can be measured as can varying degrees of under-carboxylation. The physiologic role of OCN is not clear making it difficult to determine which of the several assays for OCN is most appropriate. Most data suggest that assays detecting both the intact and major large OCN fragment are preferred, but this is not fully resolved.

The bone remodeling cycle is initiated by resorption which is rapid and lasts approximately ten days. Formation that follows is much slower lasting some ninety days. In response to therapy with an anti-resorptive drug, changes in resorption markers can be seen within 2-4 weeks of therapy while 10-12 weeks of therapy is necessary before changes in formation markers are evident. In practical terms, this is not a major concern because osteoporosis is a chronic condition where it is not essential to detect responses at 4 weeks rather than 12 weeks in most patients. There is, however, a documented medication compliance benefit from informing patients that they are responding well to therapy intended to improve their bones. Thus, there are reasons to support the use of either resorption or formation markers in osteoporosis management. Ideally, both aspects of remodeling should be evaluated, but there is little data to suggest that this provides anything but confirmatory information, and the additional expense is difficult to justify. Most of the studies relating projected rates of bone loss and initial selection of therapy have focused on resorption markers which seems most appropriate. However, the early change in formation markers have been more closely related to later changes in bone mass. Based more on opinion than fact, we favor the use of BSAP as the most specific marker of bone formation and amino-terminal telopeptide as the bone resorption marker which correlates best with changes in bone mass.

Drug Induced Metabolic Bone Disease

There are several drugs which are etiologically associated with metabolic bone disease. The majority of these offenders induce osteoporosis while those causing osteomalacia are less frequently encountered. Glucocorticoids, thyroxin, anticonvulsants, antimetabolites, and anticoagulants, in addition to alcohol, can all cause osteoporosis. Prolonged use of high doses of antacids, antidepressants, benzodiazepines, aluminum containing compounds, sodium fluoride, and etidronate all can cause osteomalacia as well.

Conclusion

The complex hormonal and non-hormonal control of serum calcium effectively maintains blood levels of this cation within a very narrow range. In primary abnormalities of bone metabolism such as osteoporosis and Paget's disease of bone, serum calcium and phophate are normal and there are demonstrable abnormalities only in the biochemical markers of osteoclast and osteoblast function. In bone diseases secondary to abnormalities in vitamin D metabolism, definite hypocalcemia is a later manifestation of disease and the bone disease is often quite advanced by this time. Metastatic bone disease causes rapid loss of bone mass with suppression of PTH and hypercalciuria. Hypercalcemia does not occur until the ability of the kidney to clear an increased filtered calcium load has been exceeded. Primary hyperparathyroidism is a resetting of the level at which serum calcium is homeostatically controlled. The skeleton is secondarily affected as a result of the increased PTH, but to a much lesser degree (usually) than in secondary hyperparathyroidism. Newer assays for calciotropic hormones and biochemical markers of bone resorption and formation have provided new insight into the pathogenesis of metabolic bone disease and have expanded the role of the clinical chemist in the evaluation and management of these patients. Increased awareness of diseases such as osteoporosis make it essential for the clinical chemist to become familiar with these new assays and to remain current with further developments. In this chapter, we have provided broad brush strokes that should stimulate the reader to delve further into the several references that accompany each section.

References

1. Parfitt AM. Morphometry of bone resorption: introduction and overview. Bone 1993;14:435-441.
2. Reichel H, Koeffler HP, Norman AW. The role of the vitamin D endocrine system in health and disease. N Engl J Med 1989;320:980-991.
3. Vorum H, Fisker K, Otagiri M, Pedersen AO, Kragh-Hansen U. Calcium ion binding to clinically relevant chemical modifications of human serum albumin. Clin Chem 1995; 41(11):1654-1661.
4. Larsson L, Ohman S. Serum ionized calcium and corrected total calcium in borderline hyperparathyroidism. Clin Chem 1978; 24(11):1962-1965.
5. Thode J, Juul-Jorgensen B, Bhatia HM, et al. Comparison of serum total calcium, albumin-corrected total calcium, and ionized calcium in 1213 patients with suspected calcium disorders [published erratum appears in Scand J Clin Lab Invest 1990; 50(1):113]. Scand J Clin Lab Invest 1989; 49(3):217-223.
6. Edelson GW, Kleerekoper M. Hypercalcemic crisis. Med Clinics N Amer 1995;79(1):79-92.
7. Lemann J. Urinary excretion of calcium, magnesium, and phosphorus. In:Favus MJ, ed. Primer on the metabolic bone diseases and disorders of mineral metabolism, 2nd ed. New York: Raven Press, 1993:50-54.
8. Okazaki R, Matsumoto T, Furukawa Y, et al. Serum intact parathyroid hormone concentration measured by a two-site immunoradiometric assay in normal subjects and patients with various parathyroid disorders. Endocrinologia Japonica. 1992;39(1):115-20.
9. Morita A, Tabata T,Koyama H, et al. A two-site immunochemiluminometric assay for intact parathyroid hormone and its clinical utility in hemodialysis patients. Clinical Nephrology. 1992;38(3):154-7.

10. Brossard JH, Cloutier M, Roy L, et al. Accumulation of a non-(1-84) molecular form of parathyroid hormone (PTH) detected by intact PTH assay in renal failure: importance in the interpretation of PTH values. J Clin Endocrinol Metab 1996; 81(11):3923-3929.

11. Henry HL, Norman AW. Vitamin D:Metabolism and biological action. Ann Rev Nutr 1984; 4:493-520.

12. Withold W, Wolff T, Degenhardt S, Reinauer H. Evaluation of a radioimmunoassay for determination of calcitriol in human sera employing a 125I-labelled tracer. European Journal of Clinical Chemistry & Clinical Biochemistry. 1995;33(12):959-63.

13. Garnero P, Delmas PD. Assessment of the serum levels of bone alkaline phosphatase with a new immunoradiometric assay in patients with metabolic bone disease. J Clin Endocrinol Metab 1993; 77(4):1046-1053.

14. Hill CS, Wolfert RL. The preparation of monoclonal antibodies which react preferentially with human bone alkaline phosphatase and not liver alkaline phosphatase. Clin Chem Acta 1986; 186:315-320.

15. McClung MR, Tou CKP, Goldstein NH, Picot C. Tiludronate therapy for Paget's disease of bone. Bone 1995; 17(suppl):493-496.

16. Prestwood KM, Pilbeam CC, Burleson JA, et al. The short term effects of conjugated estrogen on bone turnover in older women. J Clin Endocrinol Metab. 1994;79(2):366-371.

17. Chesnut CH, III, McClung MR, Ensrud KE, et al. Alendronate treatment of the postmenopausal osteoporotic woman:effect of multiple dosages on bone mass and bone remodeling. Am J Med 1995; 99:144-152.

18. Delmas PD, Wilson Detroit, Michigan, Mann KG, et al. Effect of renal function on plasma levels of bone gla-protein. J Clin Endocrinol Metab 1983; 57:1028-1030.

19. Ebeling PR, Peterson JM, Riggs BL. Role of type I procollagen propeptide assays in metabolic bone diseases. Bone Miner. 1992;17(Suppl 1):206.

20. Nordin BEC, Polley KJ. Metabolic consequences of the menopause. Calcif Tissue Int. 1987;41(Suppl 1):S1-S59.

21. Wilson PS, Kleerekoper M, Bone H, Parfitt AM. Urinary total hydroxyproline measured by HPLC: comparison of spot and timed urine collections. Clin Chem. 1990;36(2):388-389.

22. Eyre DR. New biomarkers of bone resorption [editorial]. J Clin Endocrinol Metab. 1991;74(3):470A-470C.

23. Garnero P, Delmas PD. New developments in biochemical markers for osteoporosis. Calcif Tissue Int 1996; 59(Suppl 1):S2-S9.

24. Hanson DA, Weis MAE, Bollen AM, Maslan SL, Singer FR, Eyre DR. A specific immunoassay for monitoring human bone resorption: quantitation of type I collagen cross-linked N-telopeptides in urine. J Bone Miner Res. 1992;7(11):1251-1258.

25. Risteli J, Elomaa I, Niemi S, Novamo A, Risteli L. Radioimmunoassay for the pyridinoline cross-linked carboxy-terminal telopeptide of type I collagen: a new serum marker of bone collagen degradation. Clin Chem 1993;39(4):635-640.

26. Blumsohn A, Hannon RA, Al-Dehaimi AW, Eastell R. Short-term intraindividual variability of markers of bone turnover in healthy adults [abstract 132, Sixteenth Annual ASBMR Meeting]. J Bone Miner Res 1994;9(Suppl 1).

27. Moro L, Mucelli RSP, Gazzarrini C, et al. Urinary b-1-galactosyl-O-hydroxylysine (GH) as a marker of collagen turnover of bone. Calcif Tissue Int 1988; 42:87-90.

28. Forster J, Monchik JM, Martin HF. A comparative study of serum ultrafiltrable, ionized, and total calcium in the diagnosis of primary hyperparathyroidism in patients with intermittent or no elevation in total calcium. Surgery 1988; 104(6):1137-1142.

29. Bilezikian JP. Primary Hyperparathyroidism. In:Favus MJ,ed. Primer on the metabolic bone diseases and disorders of mineral metabolism, 2nd ed. New York: Raven Press, 1993:155-159.

30. Halvorsen JF, Gautvik VT, Gautvik KM. Improved diagnosis of primary hyperparathyroidism by defining the inverse relationship between serum immunoreactive parathyroid hormone and calcium. Scand J Clin Lab Invest 1986; 46(5):435-442.

31. Nussbaum SR, Zahradnik RJ, Lavigne JR, et al. Highly sensitive two-site immunoradiometric assay of parathyrin and its clinical utility in evaluating patients with hpercalcemia. Clin Chem 1987; 33:1364-1367.

32. Brown EM, Hebert SC. Calcium-receptor-regulated parathyroid and renal function. Bone 1997; 20(4):303-309.

33. Seibel MJ, Woitge HW, Pecherstorfer M, et al. Serum immunoreactive bone sialoprotein as a new marker of bone turnover in meta-

bolic and malignant bone disease. J Clin Endocrinol Metab 1996; 81(9):3289-3294.

34. DeVernejoul MC, Kuntz D, Miravet L, et al. Bone histomorphometry in hemodialysed patients. Metab Bone Dis & Rel Res 1981; 3:175-179.

35. Hruska KA, Teitelbaum SL, Kopelman R, et al. The predictability of the histological features of uremic bone disease by noninvasive techniques. Metab Bone Dis Rel Res 1978; 1:39-44.

36. Winters RW, Graham JB, Williams TF, et al. A genetic study of familial hypophosphatemia and vitamin-D resistant rickets with a review of the literature. Medicine 1958; 37:97.

37. Hruska KA, Rolnick F. Hyperphosphatemia and hypophosphatemia. In:Favus MJ,ed. Primer on the metabolic bone diseases and disorders of mineral metabolism, 2nd ed. New York: Raven Press, 1993:213-219.

38. Roth KS, Buckalew VM Jr, Chan JCM. Renal tubular disorders. In: Gonick H (ed) Current Nephrology Yearbook, Chicago, 1985:87-117.

39. Davie MWJ, Emberson CE, Lawson DEM, et al. Low plasma 25-hydroxyvitamin D and serum calcium levels in institutionalized epileptic subjects: associated risk factors, consequences and response to treatment with vitamin D. Q J Med 1983; 52:79-91.

40. Honasoge M, Rao DS. Metabolic bone disease in gastrointestinal, hepatobiliary, and pancreatic disorders and total parenteral nutrition. Current Opinion in Rheumatology 1995; 7:249-254.

41. Colussi G, DeFerrari ME, Surean M, et al. Vitamin D metabolites and osteomalacia in the human Fanconi syndrome. Proc Eur Dial Transplant Assoc 1985; 21:756-760.

42. Drezner MK. Tumor-Induced rickets and osteomalacia. In:Favus MJ,ed. Primer on the metabolic bone diseases and disorders of mineral metabolism, 3rd ed. New York: Raven Press, 1996:319-325.

43. Mills BG, Frausto A, Singer FR, et al. Multinucleated cells formed in vitro from Paget's bone marrow express viral antigens. Bone 1994; 15:443-448.

44. Delmas PD, Meunier PJ. The management of Paget's disease of bone. N Engl J Med 1997; 336(8):558-566.

45. Meunier PJ, Salson C, Mathieu L, et al. Skeletal distribution and

biochemical parameters of Paget's disease. Clin Orthop 1987; 217:37-44.

46. Alvarez L, Guanabens N, Peris P, et al. Discriminative value of biochemical markers of bone turnover in assessing the activity of Paget's disease. J Bone Miner Res 1995; 10:458-65.
47. Bone HG, Kleerekoper M. Paget's disease of bone. J Clin Endocrinol Metab 1992; 75:1179-82.
48. Walton RJ, Preston CJ, Bartlett M, et al. Biochemical measurements in Paget's disease of bone. Eur J Clin Invest 1977; 7:37-39.
49. Tohme JF, Seibel MJ, Silverberg SJ, et al. Biochemical markers of bone metabolism. Z Rheumatol 1991; 50:133-141.
50. Uebelhart D, Gineyts E, Chapuy MCC, Delmas PD. Urinary excretion of pyridinium crosslinks: a new marker of bone resorption in metabolic bone disease. Bone Miner 1990; 8:87-96.
51. Papapoulos SE, Frolich M. Prediction of the outcome of treatment of Paget's disease of bone with bisphosphonates from short-term changes in the rate of bone resorption. Journal of Clinical Endocrinology and Metabolism 1996; 81(11):3993-3997.
52. Hamdy NAT, Papapoulos SE, Colwell A, et al. Urinary collagen crosslink excretion: a better index of bone resorption than hydroxyproline in Paget's disease of bone? Bone Miner 1993; 22:1-8.
53. Singer FR, Aldred JP, Neer RM, et al. An evaluation of antibodies and clinical resistance to salmon calcitonin. J Clin Invest 1972; 51:2331-2338.
54. Dietrich FM, Fischer JA, Bijvoet OLM. Formation of antibodies to synthetic human calcitonin during treatment of Paget's disease. Acta Endocrinol 1979; 92:468-476.
55. Altman RD, Johnston CC, Khairi MRA, et al. Influence of disodium etidronate on clinical and laboratory manifestations of Paget's disease of bone (osteitis deformans). N Engl J Med 1973; 289:1379-81.
56. Siris E, Weinstein RS, Altman R, et al. Comparative study of alendronate versus etidronate for the treatment of Paget's disease of bone. Journal of Clinical Endocrinology and Metabolism 1996; 81(3):961-967.
57. Bombassei GJ, Yocono M, Raisz LG. Effects of intravenous pamidronate therapy on Paget's disease of bone. The American Jour-

nal of the Medical Sciences 1994; 308(4):226-233.

58. McClung MR, Tou CK, Goldstein NH, et al. Tiludronate therapy for Paget's disease of bone. Bone 1995; 17:Suppl:493S-496S.

59. Chines A, Pacifici R, Avioli LV, et al. Systemic mastocytosis presenting as osteoporosis: a clinical and histomorphometric study. J Clin Endocrinol Metab 1991; 72(1):140-144.

60. Adachi JD, Bensen WG, Brown J, et al. Intermittent etidronate therapy to prevent corticosteroid-induced osteoporosis. N Engl J Med 1997; 337:382-387.

61. Brandli DW, Golde G, Greenwold M, et al. Glucocorticoid-induced osteoporosis: A cross-sectional study. Steroids 1991; 26:518-523.

62. Coindre JM, David JP, Riviere V, et al. Bone loss in hypothyroidism with hormone replacement: A histomorphometric study. Arch Intern Med 1986; 146:48-53.

63. Harrington MG, Hodkinsen PH. Anticonvulsant drugs and bone disease in the elderly. J R Soc Med 1987:80:425-427.

64. Dequeker J, Maenaut K, Verwilghen J, Westhovens R. Osteoporosis in rheumatoid arthritis. Clin Exp Rheumatol 1995; 13(Suppl 12):S21-S26.

65. Avioli LV. Heparin induced osteoporosis: An appraisal. Adv Exp Med Biol 1975; 52:375-387.

66. Akesson K, Vergnaud P, Gineyts E, et al. Impairment of bone turnover in elderly women with hip fracture. Calcif Tissue Int 1993; 53:162-169.

67. Alexeera L, Burkhardt P, Christiansen C, et al. Assessment of fracture risk and application to screening for post-menopausal osteoporosis, World Health Organization Technical Report Series 843; 1994. World Health Organization, Geneva.

68. Kleerekoper M, Edelson GW. Biochemical studies in the evaluation and management of osteoporosis: current status and future prospects. Endocrine Practice 1996;2(1):13-19.

69. Garnero P, Shih WJ, Gineyts E, Karpf DB, Delmas PD. Comparison of new biochemical markers of bone turnover in late postmenopausal osteoporotic women in response to alendronate treatment. J Clin Endocrinol Metab 1994;79:1693-1700.

70. Rosen CJ, Chesnut CH, Mallinak NJS. The predictive value of biochemical markers of bone turnover for bone mineral density in early

postmenopausal women treated with hormone replacement or calcium supplementation. J Clin Endocrinol Metab 1997; 82:1904-1910.

71. Civitelli R, Gonnelli S, Zacchei F, et al. Bone turnover in postmenopausal osteoporosis. Effect of calcitonin treatment. J Clin Invest 1988; 82:1268-1274.

72. Harris ST, Gertz BJ, Genant HK, et al. The effect of short term treatment with alendronate on vertebral density and biochemical markers of bone remodeling in early postmenopausal women. J Clin Endocrinol Metab 1993;76(6):1399-1406.

73. Garnero P, Shih WJ, Gineyts E, et al. Comparison of new biochemical markers of bone turnover in late postmenopausal osteoporotic women in response to alendronate treatment. J Clin Endocrinol Metab 1994; 79:1693-1700.

74. Ricos C, Jimenez CV, Hernandez A, et al. Biological variation in urine samples used for analyte measurements. Clin Chem 1994;40(3):472-477.

75. Schlemmer A, Hassager C, Jensen SB, Christiansen C. Marked diurnal variation in urinary excretion of pyridinium cross-links in premenopausal women. J Clin Endocrinol Metab 1992; 74(3):476-480.

76. Kleerekoper M, Wilson PS, Simpson P. Within subject variability of biochemical markers of bone remodeling in normal older women [abstract C296, Sixteenth Annual ASBMR Meeting]. J Bone Miner Res. 1994;9(Suppl 1).

77. Nielsen HK, Brixen K, Mosekilde L. Diurnal rhythm in serum activity of wheat-germ lectin-precipitable alkaline phosphatase: temporal relationships with the diurnal rhythm of serum osteocalcin. Scand J Clin Lab Invest 1990; 50(8):851-856.

78. Koyama N, Ohara K, Yokota H, et al. A one step sandwich enzyme immunoassay for y-caroboxylated osteocalcin using monoclonal antibodies. J Immunol Methods 1991;139:17-23.

79. Taylor AK, Linkart S, Moham S, et al. Multiple osteocalcin fragments in human urine and serum as detected by a midmolecule osteocalcin radioimmunoassay. J Clin Endocrinol Metab 1990; 70:467-472.

80. Garnero P, Grimaux M, Seguin P, et al. Characterization of immunoreactive forms of human osteocalcin generated in vivo and in vitro. J Bone Miner Res 1994; 9(2):255-264.

81. Harris ET, Gertz BJ, Genant HK, et al. The effect of short-term treatment with alendronate on vertebral density and biochemical markers of bone remodeling in early postmenopausal women. J Clin Endocrinol Metab 1993; 76(6):1399-1403.
82. Bohannon AD, Lyles KW. Drug-induced bone disease. Clinics in Geriatric Medicine 1994; 10(4):611-623.
83. Bikle DP, Genant HK, Lann C, et al. Bone disease in alcohol abuse. Ann Intern Med 1985; 103:42-48.
84. Cooke N, Teite L, Baum S, et al. Antacid-induced osteomalacia and nephalithiasis. Arch Intern Med 1978; 138:1007-1009.
85. Ray WA, Griffin MR. Benzodiazepines and hip fracture. JAMA 1990; 263:3260-3262.
86. Khairi MRA, Altman RD, DeRosa GP, et al. Sodium etidronate in the treatment of Paget's disease of bone: A study of long term results. Ann Intern Med 1977; 87:656-663.

6
Evaluation of Hypoglycemia & Hyperglycemia

WILLIAM E. WINTER, MD

INTRODUCTION

The body must be protected from hypoglycemia because severe acute hypoglycemia can cause coma, seizures, and even death. On the other hand, chronic hyperglycemia is toxic to blood vessels, basement membranes, and proteins that become glycated. Therefore the body must maintain the level of energy currency (glucose) in the blood stream within narrow limits. This is a challenging task because the biochemical demands for glucose throughout the body can vary tremendously. Whereas there are four hormones specifically designed to raise glucose concentrations in the blood stream (epinephrine, glucagon, cortisol, and growth hormone), there is only one hormone designed to specifically lower glucose concentrations: insulin. This chapter addresses the etiologies and diagnostic workups for hypo- and hyperglycemia

I) Clinical Symptoms Of Hypoglycemia

In routine medical practice, hypoglycemia (low blood glucose) is commonly encountered in the immediate neonatal period (especially in premature infants and infants born to diabetic mothers) and in insulin-treated diabetic patients who take excessive doses of insulin, skip meals, and/or exercise more than usual. Acute hypoglycemia produces adrenergic symptoms (e.g., tachycardia, palpitations, pounding heart, sweating, tremulousness, anxiety, nervousness, feeling cold, and sweating) and neuroglycopenia [low blood glucose in the brain: decreased consciousness, tiredness or drowsiness, faintness, confusion, blurred or double vision, hemiparesis, behavioral changes, dizziness, paresthesias (pins and needles feelings), incoordination, slurred speech, hunger, headache].

II) Fasting Hypoglycemia Versus Reactive Hypoglycemia

Fasting (postabsorptive) hypoglycemia may occur in the morning prior to eating, between meals, or with exercise. Fasting hypoglycemia usually implies a serious condition that requires thorough medical evaluation. Reactive hypoglycemia is also referred to as "postprandial" or "stimulative" hypoglycemia. This form of reputed hypoglycemia usually does *not* imply a serious disorder. The hypothesis behind "reactive" (or food stimulated) hypoglycemia is that excessive release of insulin follows a large glucose load and causes hypoglycemia several hours after eating. Many patients with symptoms of reactive hypoglycemia regularly miss meals and/or do not eat a balanced diet (e.g.., ~55-60% carbohydrate, ~15% protein, ~≤30% fat).

The diagnosis of reactive hypoglycemia is sometimes pursued by performing a 5 hour oral glucose tolerance test (OGTT). When patients with hypoglycemic-like symptoms manifest a glucose of <40 mg/dL in the later stages of the OGTT, reactive hypoglycemia is diagnosed. However, ≥10% of adults display glucose values of <50 mg/dL at 3 or more hours after an oral glucose challenge. In such general population studies, there has been no correlation between the adrenergic symptoms of reactive hypoglycemia and glucose values <50 mg/dL 3 to 5 hours after the oral glucose load. For this reason, most endocrinologists do *not* consider reactive hypoglycemia to be a disease (1,2). *Clinicians should therefore be discouraged from performing 5 hour OGTTs.* Successful treatment of reactive hypoglycemia involves achieving healthy eating patterns and regular meals.

The only hypoglycemic disorder that is really "reactive" involves the "dumping" syndrome where food rapidly transits from the stomach to the small intestine and large amounts of glucose are rapidly absorbed. Subsequently, there is a surge of insulin release that does in fact lead to true "reactive" hypoglycemia. This form of "reactive" hypoglycemia can be treated with smaller, more frequent meals.

III) Diagnosis Of Hypoglycemia

The diagnosis of hypoglycemia is established when three criteria ("Whipple's triad") are documented: 1) symptoms compatible with hypoglycemia are substantiated; 2) there is laboratory confirmation of a low blood glucose concentration at the time of symptoms (serum or plasma glucose <45 mg/dL), and 3) symptoms are relieved promptly with the rapid administration of glucose. Because self-blood-glucose-monitoring (SBGM) systems are not accurate at values <40-60 mg/dL, the glucose determination must be performed in the central laboratory. However, SBGM can be used by the patient at home when the clinician wants to determine (preliminarily) whether the patient has any biochemical evidence suggestive of hypoglycemia prior to beginning an involved workup for suspected hypoglycemia.

IV) Biochemical Definition Of Hypoglycemia

Hypoglycemia is biochemically defined as a *venous* whole blood glucose of <40 mg/dL or a *venous* plasma or serum glucose of <45 mg/dL. Some references set a cutoff for hypoglycemia as a serum or plasma glucose <40 mg/dL. Because glucose concentrations are not affected by changes in the hematocrit, plasma or serum are the preferred specimens for glucose analysis when analyzed rapidly. Although newborns, especially premature infants, commonly display glucose values of 20-40 mg/dL or less, these values are considered to be potentially harmful. Therefore, the definition of hypoglycemia described above applies to individuals regardless of age.

Pseudohypoglycemia occurs when the measured blood glucose is artifactually depressed because of delayed analysis. Because cellular elements of the blood stream (e.g., white blood cells and to a lesser degree red blood cells) consume glucose, unless samples are to be assayed within 1 hour of being drawn, blood should be drawn into gray top tubes containing NaF to inhibit glycolysis. Without the addition of NaF, serum or plasma glucose will fall by ~5-7% per hour. High white blood cell counts (e.g., chronic myelocytic leukemia) produce more rapid rates of decline in blood glucose. Samples placed in NaF tubes will be stable at room temperature for 24 hours.

V) Causes Of Hypoglycemia

In the absence of a recognized cause of hypoglycemia (e.g., an infant born to a diabetic mother or a diabetic patient who took a known overdose of insulin), the initial differentiation to establish is whether the patient has hyperinsulinemic hypoglycemia or nonhyperinsulinemic hypoglycemia. Assuming that hypoglycemia has been biochemically confirmed, the age of the patient has a major effect on the likely causes of hypoglycemia. Therefore the age of the patient influences the tests that are actually run. For example, *in individuals that first develop hypoglycemia after ages 4 or 5 years, studies in search of inborn errors of metabolism should not be pursued.* Table 1 provides a listing of causes of hypoglycemia. Within each age group, the etiologies of hypoglycemia are classified as to their frequency, e.g., +++: very common; ++: common; +: occasional; -: rare; - - -: does not occur.

Table 1: Causes of Hypoglycemia by Age: Relative Frequency as Causes of Hypoglycemia

	NEONATE	CHILD	ADULT
Hyperinsulinism	++	++	+++
Drugs	+	+++	+++
Hormone Deficiency	++	++	+
Inborn Errors	++	+	-
Liver disease	++	++	++
Renal disease	-	-	-
Extrapancreatic neoplasm	-	-	+
Critical or severe illness	+++	++	+
Neonatal hypoglycemia	+++	- - -	- - -
Ketotic hypoglycemia	- - -	++	- - -
Severe malnutrition	+	+	+

VI) Diagnostic Workup For Hypoglycemia

A) Evaluation of Acute Hypoglycemia

Should the patient suffer an acute episode of hypoglycemia (e.g., the patient arrives in the emergency room in coma and is found to be hypoglycemic), table 2 lists the studies that should be considered. If possible, more than one sample should be obtained at this time (e.g., the initial sample and a sample drawn just before IV glucose or glucagon are administered). Tests for the evaluation of hypoglycemia can be divided into *routine* **versus** *optional*, and those tests that *should be obtained at the time of acute hypoglycemia* **versus** *those tests that need not be obtained at the time of acute hypoglycemia*. The optional tests to be pursued are dependent upon the patient's age, history, physical examination, and likely cause of hypoglycemia depending upon the specific clinical situation. For example, if in the initial evaluation the patient is found to have liver failure, other causes of hypoglycemia are less likely and need not be immediately pursued. These guidelines for obtaining samples also apply to prolonged fasts.

In the absence of an acute hypoglycemic episode, the best time to *screen* for hypoglycemia is in the morning after an overnight fast. Plasma glucose values of <45 mg/dL are consistent with hypoglycemia, while plasma glucose concentrations of 45-60 mg/dL are suggestive of hypoglycemia. In either case, further evaluation is indicated (e.g., a prolonged fast). When hypoglycemia is a serious clinical consideration, several fasting blood glucose determinations are warranted before hypoglycemia is excluded. Plasma glucose concentrations >60 mg/dL are normal and when present on several occasions (in the absence of any values ≤60 mg/dL) rule against fasting hypoglycemia.

B) Prolonged Fasts in the Evaluation of Hypoglycemia

A **prolonged fast** lasting up to 72 hours may be required to determine whether of not hypoglycemia actually occurs. In children with ketotic hypoglycemia, fasting for as little as 8 hours may precipitate hypoglycemia. This probably reflects the limited biochemical abilities of children to maintain normoglycemia because of their proportionately smaller muscle mass and higher ratio of brain size to liver size (e.g., glucose consumer to glucose producer ratio compared to adults). Prolonged fasts are performed in hospital so that purported symptoms and signs of hypoglycemia can be carefully recorded, glucose concentrations can be regularly measured, blood samples can be obtained for analysis, intravenous glucose is available for emergency administration, and intravenous glucagon can be administered

Table 2: Biochemical Studies in the Evaluation of Hypoglycemia

TEST	INDICATION
Routine measurements in adults and children at the time of acute hypoglycemia	
Plasma glucose	Measured to diagnose hypoglycemia; decreased value is necessary for the diagnosis of hypoglycemia
ßHB (and/ or) urine ketones	Assessment of ketosis; hyperinsulinism can suppress ketosis
Routine measurements in infants and young children at the time of acute hypoglycemia	
Lactic acid	Assessment for lactic acidosis; measurement in adults is optional
Urine reducing substances	Measured to exclude certain inborn errors of carbohydrate metabolism; measure in all infants (eg., ≤2 years): measure at a time when the infant is on their normal diet
Optional measurements at the time of acute hypoglycemia	
Drug screen/Ethanol	Performed to rule out intoxication; perform blood/urine screening when intoxication can not be otherwise excluded; screen for sulfonylureas when indicated
Insulin	Measured to rule out hyperinsulinism; hold sample for insulin measurement if indicated
Cortisol*	Measured to rule out hypocortisolism; hold sample for cortisol measurement if indicated
Human Growth Hormone (hGH)	Measured to rule out hGH deficiency; hold sample for hGH measurement if indicated
C-peptide	Measured to confirm that hyperinsulinism is endogenous; C-peptide is elevated in insulinoma and sulfonylurea toxicity, with exogenous insulin administration, C-peptide is suppressed
Branched chain amino acids	Measured to document the biochemical effects of hyperinsulinism; rarely needed; helpful in confirming "functional" hyperinsulin ism** when insulin levels are low
Free fatty acids (FFAs)	Measured to document the biochemical effects of hyperinsulinism or suspected fatty acid oxidation disorders (FAOD)
Urine dicarboxylic acids	Measured when an aminoacidopathy or FAOD are suspected
Arterial blood gases[1]	Measured to assess acid/base balance; acidosis is common in many disorders that cause hypoglycemia
HCO_3-, Cl-, urine pH	Measured to assess acid/base balance; acidosis is common in many disorders that cause hypoglycemia
Routine measurements not required at the time of acute hypoglycemia	
Liver function[2]	Measured to rule out: liver disease
Renal function[3]	Measured to rule out: kidney disease
Urinalysis	Measured to assess renal disease
Optional measurements not required at the time of acute hypoglycemia	
Thyroid studies[4]	Measured to rule out thyroid dysfunction; measure when thyroid disease is clinically suspected
Serum/plasma amino acids	Measured to rule out amino acidopathy
Uric acid	Measured when inborn errors of metabolism are a consideration; elevated when lactate is elevated
Cholesterol/Triglycerides	Measured when inborn errors of metabolism are a consideration; elevated in certain glycogen stoarge diseases
Creatine kinase	Measured when myopathy is suspected; elevated in certain glycogen storage diseases
Carnitine	Measured when FAOD is suspected; low in cases of carnitine deficiency

**Rule out: hypopituitarism; **: for example: IGF-II producing tumor, agonistic anti-insulin receptor autoantibody; 1: pH, pO_2, pCO_2; 2: ALT, AST, alkaline phosphatase, total bilirubin, direct bilirubin, albumin, total protein, consider protime (PT); 3: creatinine, BUN; 4) TSH, T4, T3, T3RU/T-Uptake, or TSH and unbound T4.*

at the termination of the fast. During the fast, the subject is npo (nothing by mouth) except for free access to water.

At the beginning of the prolonged fast (before retiring for sleep), an intravenous line is introduced into a vein of sufficient size so that blood can be periodically withdrawn for analysis. The line is flushed with a heparinized saline solution (e.g., 100 units/mL) and clamped. Prior to drawing subsequent samples, 3 to 5 mL of blood are withdrawn to clear the line of the flush solution (e.g., drawing a "blank").

Blood glucose must be drawn as a baseline value at the beginning of the fast. Because adrenergic symptoms of hypoglycemia can become attenuated in some individuals who suffer chronic and recurrent hypoglycemia, during the fast the blood glucose must be measured regularly (e.g., every 4 hours) by the central laboratory. Between these 4 hour measurements, finger-stick capillary glucose can be measured with a meter to monitor the course of the fast. If any of the capillary glucose values show a significant decline (e.g., decrease of ≥10 mg/dL), a confirmatory venous glucose can be drawn from the indwelling catheter. Recall that capillary glucose values require correction to serum levels (capillary glucose x 1.15 = serum glucose) as capillary and whole blood glucose values are ~15% lower than venous serum glucose values.

During the fast all urine samples are tested for ketones. Once the blood glucose drops *below 60 mg/dL*, venous draws can be increased to every two hours. The fast is continued until frank symptoms of hypoglycemia are present (see Tables 1 and 2) or the venous glucose is persistently <45 mg/dL (e.g., for at least 30 minutes). If this does *not* occur by 72 hours, fasting hypoglycemia is excluded and further studies are not indicated.

Once symptoms of hypoglycemia initially occur or the venous glucose initially falls below 45 mg/dL, blood should be drawn for clinical studies (Table 2). This is a critical time for sampling when the laboratory results are most informative. Blood should be drawn again ~30 minutes later and the glucose repeated. Because the inclusion or exclusion of hyperinsulinism is key to the differential diagnosis of hypoglycemia, insulin should essentially always be measured (see below).

At the termination of the fast if biochemical hypoglycemia is documented, intravenous glucagon (1 mg or 0.03 mg/kg, minimum dose in children is usually 0.5 mg) is administered IV. Blood for glucose measurement is drawn ~every 10 to 15 minutes for up to 45 minutes and blood is again stored for future analyses as described above. Obviously, the tests actually run depend upon the age of the patient, clinical history, physical examination, and clinical suspicion. The laboratory should be able to process and hold specimens until the physician decides which studies are required.

VII) Testing Strategy For Evaluation Of Hypoglycemia

In the differential diagnosis of hypoglycemia, the first diagnostic assessment concerns whether hyperinsulinism is present or absent at the time of hypoglycemia. This divides the etiologies of hypoglycemia into *hyperinsulinemic hypoglycemia* (Figure 1) and *nonhyperinsulinemic hypoglycemia* (Figure 2).

Figure 1.Hyperinsulinemic Hypoglycemia

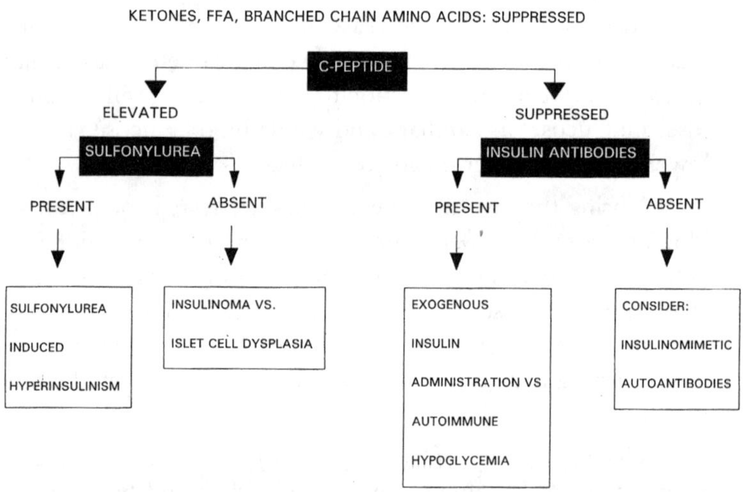

FIGURE 2. NONHYPERINSULINEMIC HYPOGLYCEMIA

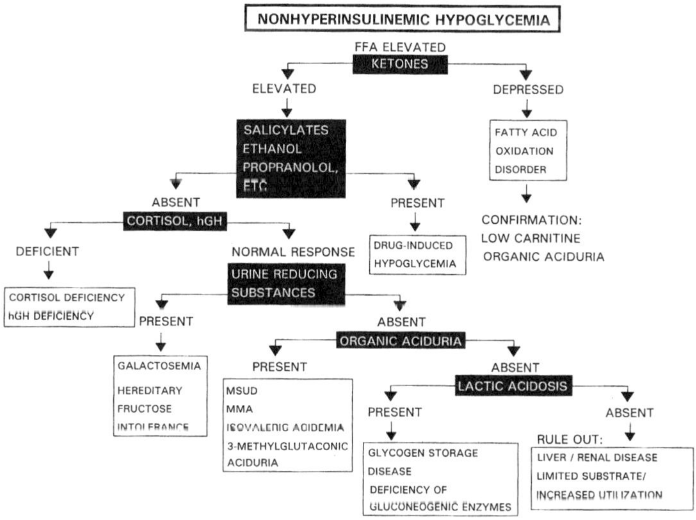

A) Hypoglycemia syndromes with Hyperinsulinism or Functional Hyperinsulinism

To determine if hyperinsulinemic hypoglycemia is present, the clinician must assess two aspects of the patient's presentation: 1) the insulin concentration relative to the glucose concentration and 2) whether other biochemical findings (e.g., urine ketones, ßHB, FFAs, branched chain amino acids) are consistent with hyperinsulinism. "Functional" hyperinsulinism occurs when the insulin concentration is inappropriately elevated for the blood glucose concentration or when there is an insulin surrogate [e.g., elevated IGF-II (insulin like growth factor II) or an agonistic anti-insulin receptor autoantibody (insulinomimetic autoantibody)]. Some clinicians find that calculating the insulin to glucose ratio is helpful in diagnosing hyperinsulinism. If the insulin to glucose ratio is >0.25-0.30 (100 x mIU/mg), hyperinsulinism is diagnosed. However great care must be applied with reference to the specific insulin assay that is used. For example in a recent comparison in my laboratory, the insulin assay on a popular random access automated analyzer gave insulin concentrations 40% less those determined by a popular radioimmunoassay (RIA) kit. Therefore to compensate for this difference, clinicians would need to modify the insulin : glucose ratio cutoff to 0.18 from 0.30 (e.g., 0.30 x 0.60 = 0.18 with 0.60 being the slope of the automated analyzer insulin versus the RIA insulin). An elevated proinsulin level or proinsulin to total insulin ratio in the face of hypoglycemia can also suggest hyperinsulinism. An amended insulin to glucose ratio was proposed in the 1970s: ([insulin] x 100) ÷ (glucose -30 mg/dL) (abnormal >50). However some authors believe that the best assessment for hyperinsulinism is the measurement of absolute insulin concentration during hypoglycemia. If the glucose is <40 mg/dL, the insulin concentration should be <6 mU/mL. In one report, this later approach identified more than 99% of hyperinsulinemic individuals. Malignant insulinomas may be recognized by an elevated hCG concentration.

With functional hyperinsulinism, the following laboratory results are usually observed:

- urine *negative* for ketones
- *normal* ßHB[4] (ßHB is not elevated)
- *normal* FFA concentrations (FAAs are not elevated)
- *normal* branched chain amino acids[5] (branched chain amino acids are not elevated)

These findings reflect the suppressive effect of hyperinsulinism on the generation of alternative fuels (e.g., ketones) and the suppressive effect of hyperinsulinism on the liberation of amino acids from muscle (e.g., branched chain amino acids) as substrate for gluconeogenesis. FFA and branched chain amino acid determinations will usually be available only at referral laboratories. *The absence of urine ketones and normal ßHB in the face of hypoglycemia should alert the clinician and laboratorian to the possibility of actual or functional hyperinsulinism.* However by itself, the presence of urine ketones does *not* exclude hyperinsulinism. Lactic acidosis or elevated lactate does not occur as part of the hyperinsulinism syndromes. As will be discussed, lactic acidosis is seen with certain inborn errors of metabolism involving, for example, defective gluconeogenesis or glycogenolysis (e.g., glycogen storage disease).

Another clinical aid in making the diagnosis of hyperinsulinism is the blood glucose response to glucagon administration. This is usually done at the completion of a period of fasting when hypoglycemia has been confirmed or with acute hypoglycemia if glucagon is available for emergency administration. When hyperinsulinism is present, exogenous glucagon administered in a pharmacologic dose (e.g., 1 mg IM or IV) reverses hyperinsulinemic inhibition of glycogenolysis (as well as gluconeogenesis) and promotes rapid glycogenolysis raising the blood glucose ≥40 mg/dL within ~45 minutes (3). With other causes of nonhyperinsulinemic hypoglycemia, blood glucose response to glucagon is <40 mg/dL and can be delayed or absent.

A1a) Elevated Insulin to Glucose Ratio with Elevated C-peptide

When the pancreatic beta cell is the source of the hyperinsulinism (e.g., elevated C-peptide and insulin) (4), the beta cell may be functioning *autonomously* (e.g., insulinoma) or the beta cell may be *stimulated* to oversecrete insulin by drugs or, rarely, by autoantibodies. The differential diagnosis of autonomous beta cell hyperfunction in neonates includes transient hyperinsulinism associated with small for gestational age (SGA) infants, or transient hyperinsulinism secondary to exposure to maternal hyperglycemia [e.g., infant of diabetic mother (IDM)], or erythroblastosis fetalis. When hypoglycemia is prolonged beyond the first or second week of life, islet dysplasia (dysmaturity, e.g., nesidioblastosis) or congenital disorders (e.g., Beckwith Wiedemann syndrome: clinical diagnosis: macroglossia and omphalocele) should be considered. Endogenous hyperinsulinism in children can be caused by islet cell dysplasia or uncommonly by insulinoma. Endogenous hyperinsulinism in adults is caused by insulinoma.

Even in adults, insulinomas are uncommon with a yearly incidence reported at 1:1,000,000 to 1:1,250,000. There is no strict sex bias (60:40; female: male ratio). Most patients with insulinoma are 40 to 60 years old. Ten percent of insulinomas occur in patients less than age 20 and 10% of cases occur in patients greater than age 60. In ~4% of cases, insulinoma is associated with the multiple endocrine neoplasia (MEN) syndrome type I (i.e., tumors of the pituitary, pancreatic islets, and parathyroid glands). With MEN type I, insulinoma may be multifocal. Multiple insulinomas are found in 6% to 10% of affected patients. The majority of children (and some adults) do not have discrete islet cell tumors but display islet hypertrophy.

Ten percent of insulinomas are malignant as identified by the presence of metastases to peripancreatic lymph nodes and/or the liver. Only 2% of insulinomas are extrapancreatic (e.g., located in the duodenal wall or porta hepatis). Patients with insulinoma may have symptoms for 2 weeks to 20 years before the diagnosis is made. *Following drug-induced hypoglycemia, insulinoma is the most common cause of hypoglycemia in adults.*

When the insulin to glucose ratio is high and C-peptide is elevated, drug-induced hyperinsulinism should also be considered. The most common types of drugs to produce hyperinsulinism are the sulfonylureas. To a far lesser extent, quinine and pentamidine have reportedly caused hypoglycemia. Recognize also that pentamidine can cause glucose intolerance. When sulfonylurea use can not be excluded, toxicologic testing of the urine for sulfonylureas is indicated. Drugs that stimulate insulin secretion by the beta cell are fairly common causes of hypoglycemia in the adult population.

Alternatively the beta cell may be stimulated to oversecrete insulin by spontaneous anti-beta cell agonist autoantibodies (e.g., "Graves disease of the beta cell"). In practical terms, this condition is mentioned only for completeness recognizing that this is a diagnosis of exclusion, and indeed, such cases would be reportable in the medical literature because of their rarity.

A1b) Elevated Insulin to Glucose Ratio with Suppressed C-peptide

Assuming that hyperinsulinism is present, *measuring C-peptide at the time of hypoglycemia will determine whether the source of the insulin is endogenous* (e.g., from the pancreatic beta cells: C-peptide elevated) *or exogenous* [e.g., from insulin injection or insulin antibodies (autoimmune hypoglycemia): C-peptide low or absent]. With surreptitious insulin injection, the insulin to glucose ratio at the time of hypoglycemia is elevated yet C-peptide is not detectable because C-peptide is absent from commercial insulin preparations.

Rare in the U.S. but common in Japan is the autoimmune hypoglycemia syndrome. Similar to clandestine administration of exogenous insulin, with autoimmune hypoglycemia the insulin to glucose ratio could be elevated while C-peptide is not elevated. In this disorder, spontaneous autoantibodies to insulin develop and bind large quantities of insulin in the circulation. At certain times, glucose intolerance can be present when free insulin concentrations are deficient. At other times, insulin will be released from the insulin autoantibodies at a rate inappropriate for metabolic needs causing hypoglycemia. *Thus the key to recognizing exogenous insulin administration and autoimmune hypoglycemia is an elevated insulin to glucose ratio at the time of hypoglycemia, absent or low C-peptide, and the finding of antibodies to insulin.* With endogenous hyperinsulinism, the molar insulin/C-peptide ratio is <1. With exogenous hyperinsulinism, the molar insulin/C-peptide ratio is ≥ 1 (5).

A2) Functional Hyperinsulinism: Biochemical Findings Compatible with Hyperinsulinism with Suppressed Insulin Concentrations

In the face of confirmed hypoglycemia when ketogenesis is absent (negative urine ketones, normal ßHB) and branched chain amino acids are normal, *and the insulin to glucose ratio is not elevated*, *insulin surrogates* as causes of hypoglycemia must be contemplated. Note that insulin surrogates (other than insulinomimetic autoantibodies) are not included in Figure 1 but can, nonetheless, be diagnosed based upon this present discussion. Mesothelial tumors that secrete IGF-II should be considered (6). At high concentrations, IGF-II binds to the insulin receptor causing hypoglycemia which, in turn, suppresses pancreatic insulin secretion. High IGF-II also suppresses growth hormone (GH) which in turn leads to low concentrations of circulating IGF-I.

Insulinomimetic autoantibodies have been described above. Because of autoantibody binding to the insulin receptor, insulinomimetic autoantibodies may actually impede the clearance of any endogenously secreted insulin which may occasionally elevate insulin concentrations. Insulinomimetic autoantibody measurements are available only on a research basis.

B) Nonhyperinsulinemic Hypoglycemia

If absolute or functional hyperinsulinism is excluded, the results of other tests drawn at the time of hypoglycemia (or during the workup) are reviewed in evaluating the other potential etiologies of hypoglycemia (Figure 2). It should be emphasized that sufficient volume and types of specimens of blood and urine should be obtained at the time of acute hypoglycemia to perform all of the needed tests.

The causes of nonhyperinsulinemic hypoglycemia (Table 3) can be divided into those conditions where ketones and FFAs are *both* elevated *versus* those conditions where ketones are *depressed* and FFAs are *elevated* (disorders of fatty acid oxidation). This contrasts with the condition discussed previously, with absolute or functional hyperinsulinism [e.g., true hyperinsulinism, or insulin surrogates (e.g., elevated IGF-II or insulinomimetic autoantibody)], in which ketones (e.g., urine ketones and ßHB) and FFAs are *both suppressed*. The etiologies listed in Table 3 can be directly assessed by laboratory analysis and history.

Table 3: Causes of Nonhyperinsulinemic Hypoglycemia

ELEVATED KETONES AND FFAS	
Drugs	
	Ethanol
	Salicylates
	Propranolol
Hormone Deficiency	
	Growth hormone (GH) deficiency
	Adrenal insufficiency
	Hypopituitarism
	Thyroid dysfunction
	Pheochromocytoma
Inborn Errors of Metabolism	
	Carbohydrate disorders
	Amino acidopathies
Liver disease	
Renal disease	
Substrate limited/Increased utilization	
	Critical or severe illness
	Neonatal hypoglycemia
	Severe malnutrition
	Non-IGF-II secreting extrapancreatic neoplasms
	Ketotic hypoglycemia
SUPPRESSED KETONES AND ELEVATED FFA	
Disorders of Fatty Acid Metabolism	
	Systemic carnitine deficiency
	Carnitine palmityl transferase (CPT) deficiency
	Acyl-CoA dehydrogenase deficiency
	Glutaric aciduria type II
	HMG CoA lyase deficiency

B1) Drugs as Causes of Hypoglycemia

A history of drug ingestion must always be sought in cases of hypoglycemia (Figure 2). If ethanol poisoning is a clinical consideration, the blood ethanol (alcohol) concentration should be measured at the time the patient is hypoglycemic. Salicylate poisoning can produce hypoglycemia from liver dysfunction. Salicylates can be tested for in the urine or a serum salicylate level can be measured. Propranolol, as detected by thin layer chromatography, can produce hypoglycemia by blocking the metabolic effects of epinephrine.

B2) Endocrinopathies as Causes of Hypoglycemia

ACTH and GH deficiency can be isolated pituitary defects or, more commonly, they can coexist as components of panhypopituitarism. Primary adrenocortical insufficiency is recognized clinically because of hypoglycemia, hyponatremia, hyperkalemia, acidosis, and shock (e.g., Addisonian crisis) (7). Cortisol concentrations of <20 mg/dL at the time of hypoglycemia are suggestive of ACTH or primary adrenal insufficiency. Growth hormone deficiency is suggested by a GH concentration of <7-10 ng/mL (depending upon the specific GH immunoassay) during a hypoglycemic episode.

Thyroid dysfunction (e.g., hypothyroidism) is a rare cause of hypoglycemia and should be pursued only *when* there is a clinical suspicion of thyroid disease. Patients with pheochromocytoma are unlikely to be initially diagnosed because of hypoglycemia. The diagnosis of pheochromocytoma is considered when there is a history of episodic and/or severe hypertension. Epinephrine deficiency and glucagon deficiency are essentially only theoretical causes of hypoglycemia that do not justify measurements of either catecholamines or glucagon during periods of hypoglycemia.

B3) Carbohydrate and Amino Acid Inborn Errors of Metabolism Causing Hypoglycemia

These rare disorders occur almost exclusively in newborns and infants (Figure 2). While hypoglycemia may be an important clinical aspect of these diseases, other clinical findings such as seizures, acidosis, lethargy, or liver disease are the usual initial complaints.

B3a) Disorders of Carbohydrate Metabolism

B3ai) Galactosemia and Hereditary Fructose Intolerance

These two categories are grouped together because nonglucose carbohydrate excretion in the urine produces a *positive urine test for reducing substances but a negative result on urine glucose dipstick testing* (e.g., glucose oxidase method) (Figure 2). The clinical findings in galactosemia include early onset cataracts, hepatomegaly, liver dysfunction or failure (as evidenced in hyperbilirubinemia), mental retardation (when untreated), and failure to thrive (e.g., failure to grow). Galactosemia is clinically recognized because of the above symptoms and signs although hypoglycemia can be observed on *rare* occasions. Galactosemia is not a single disease entity. Three inborn errors which are inherited in a autosomal recessive pattern, galactokinase deficiency, galactose-1-phosphate uridyl transferase and uridine diphosphate galactose-4-epimerase deficiency can cause galactosemia. The galactose-1-phosphate uridyl transferase assay measurement in red blood cells is available in reference laboratories.

Hereditary fructose intolerance (aldolase B deficiency) is manifested when fructose [that is part of sucrose (table sugar)] is first introduced into the diet at ~3 to 6 months of age. This differs from galactosemia where disease onset occurs shortly after birth. Hypoglycemia and metabolic derangements following fructose ingestion are short lived. However without fructose restriction, hepatic and kidney failure may develop leading to death. Infants can display poor feeding, vomiting, failure to thrive, hepatomegaly, jaundice (due to liver dysfunction), or hemorrhage (due to decreased clotting factor production).

B3aii) The glycogen storage diseases

In the glycogen storage diseases (GSDs) types I, III, and VI, there is a defect in the breakdown of glycogen to glucose leading to increased hepatic glycogen stores, subsequent hepatomegaly, and hypoglycemia. Insulin secretion is suppressed, glucagon concentrations are elevated, hyperlipidemia is common, and growth retardation results when hypoglycemia and lactic acidosis are not prevented. The initial complaint is usually hepatomegaly with or without hypoglycemia.

The most severe form of GSD is von Gierke's disease (*GSD type I*) which results from a deficiency of glucose-6-phosphatase (type Ia disease) or a defect in the glucose-6-phosphatase transport (glucose-6-phosphate translocase) system (type Ib disease). Characteristic laboratory findings include fasting hypoglycemia, lactic acidosis, hyperuricemia, hypertriglyceridemia, and hypercholesterolemia. There is *no* increase in the blood glucose concentration in response to glucagon injection.

Amylo-1,6 glucosidase transfers 3 to 4 glucose units in 1 → 4 linkages from the branch chain to the main chain leaving a single glucose residue in the branched chain in a 1 → 6 linkage. Subsequently, free glucose is released by the action of amylo-1,6 glucosidase upon the 1 → 6 linkage. Without normal amylo-1,6 glucosidase activity, after some hours of fasting, glycogen can no longer be degraded and hypoglycemia may ensue. This problem causes *GSD type III*. In addition to hepatomegaly (which may resolve after puberty), there is muscular weakness in adulthood. The biochemical findings are similar to, although less severe than, GSD type I. Creatine kinase (CK) may be elevated because of myopathy. For some hours after eating, blood glucose concentrations will increase after glucagon injection in GSD type III.

GSD type VI (Hers disease) results from a deficiency of liver phosphorylase or phosphorylase b kinase. Similar to GSD type I, muscle is not affected in GSD type VI. Hepatomegaly is recognized. Only mild hypoglycemia may be observed. Deficiency of glycogen synthase (*GSD type* O) is very rare.

B3aiii) Defects in Gluconeogenic Enzymes

In addition to glucose-6-phosphatase, *pyruvate carboxylase (PC), phosphoenol pyruvate carboxykinase (PEPCK), and fructose 1,6-bisphosphatase* are required for gluconeogenesis. With a deficiency of any of these enzymes, glucose can not be regenerated from lactic acid causing hypoglycemia and lactic acidosis (i.e., the Cori cycle is interrupted).

B3b) Amino Acidopathies with Associated Hypoglycemia

Similar to many of the defects described under disorders of the fatty acid oxidation and gluconeogenic enzyme deficiencies, *amino acidopathies often precipitate overwhelming illness in the first days of life frequently noted as acidosis and organic aciduria* (Figure 2). While hypoglycemia may be present in all of these disorders (e.g., maple syrup urine disease, methyl malonic aciduria, isovaleric acidemia, 3-methylglutaconic aciduria), hypoglycemia is not the sole initial complaint and hypoglycemia is just one aspect of these systemic, metabolic disorders.

B4) Liver and Renal Disorders as Causes of Hypoglycemia

Hepatic or renal disease as contributors to hypoglycemia are easily assessed (Figure 2) by the liver and kidney function tests mentioned. However, renal and hepatic disorders as causes of hypoglycemia should be considered diagnoses of exclusion (e.g., other causes of hypoglycemia must be excluded before hypoglycemia can be attributed strictly to liver or renal disease).

B5) Limited Substrate/Increased Utilization as Causes of Hypoglycemia

The common theme in these disorders is increased demand for glucose (often because of critical illness) and/or decreased hepatic ability to produce glucose (Figure 2). *Sepsis* in neonates or child may produce hypoglycemia. The mechanism of hypoglycemia in *cyanotic congenital heart disease* is unclear. *Newborn infants*, especially premature infants, are at high risk for hypoglycemia based on liver immaturity, high caloric demands (e.g., countering cold stress), limited or no caloric intake immediately following birth, limited amino acid substrate for gluconeogenesis (e.g., minimal muscle mass), limited ability to generate ketones, and an increased proportion of brain size to liver size further increasing glucose demands. With *severe malnutrition* (i.e., kwashiorkor), there is depletion of all energy resources needed for glucose generation (e.g., very low muscle mass) and ketone body generation (e.g., exhausted supply of triglycerides from adipose tissue).

The non-IGF-II secreting *extrapancreatic neoplasms* are theorized to anaerobically consume glucose at high rates producing hypoglycemia and elevated lactate concentrations.

Ketotic hypoglycemia is a clinical diagnosis based upon the development of hypoglycemia, ketonuria, and vomiting after only modest durations of fasting (e.g., overnight) in otherwise healthy children between ages 18 months and 6 years of age. There are *no* inborn errors of metabolism in this condition. These children are often male and were small for gestational age at birth.

B6) Disorders of Fatty Acid Oxidation

Similar to amino acidopathies and carbohydrate disorders that cause hypoglycemia, disorders of fatty acid oxidation present in the newborn period or during infancy. These disorders lead to a deficiency of ketone body production. With ketone body deficiency, the sole source of energy during fasting becomes glucose. With increased glucose demands during fasting (because alternative fuels are not available), glucose production does not keep pace with glucose demand and hypoglycemia ensues.

When ketone production is *low* (e.g., absent urine ketones, normal ßHB) and FFAs are *elevated*, a disorder of fatty acid oxidation is suggested. *Carnitine* should be measured as carnitine concentrations are frequently low in these syndromes. When fatty acids can not be oxidized by ß-oxidation, omega-oxidation occurs producing dicarboxylic acids that are excreted in the urine.

VIII) Summary Of The Evaluation Of Hypoglycemia

The potential causes of hypoglycemia are legion. The differential diagnosis and laboratory evaluation of hypoglycemia should be assessed according to the patient's age, history, and physical examination. Figures 1 and 2 provide a reasonable approach to sorting out these disorders. A specific diagnosis must always be sought so that proper therapy can be pursued.

IX) Differential Diagnosis Of Hyperglycemia

The American Diabetes Association (ADA) has recently defined fasting hyperglycemia as fasting plasma glucose levels $\geq$126 mg/dL. The upper limit of the reference range for fasting plasma glucose remains <110. When the fasting plasma glucose is between 110 and 125 mg/dL, a state of "impaired fasting glucose" (IFG) exists. Such individuals with IFG are at high risk to develop diabetes mellitus in the future. Hyperglycemia can be classified as transient (acute) or sustained (chronic). Chronic hyperglycemia constitutes diabetes mellitus. Causes of transient hyperglycemia include:

- Significant degrees of metabolic stress (secondary to elevations in the anti-insulin "stress" hormones: glucagon, epinephrine, cortisol and growth hormone)
  Myocardial infarction
  Burns
  Acute, severe illness
- Medications used for short durations of time (e.g., only days to weeks)
  Glucocorticoids (an anti-insulin "stress" hormone)
  Catecholamines (an anti-insulin "stress" hormone)
  Encainide (suppression of insulin secretion)
  Growth hormone (an anti-insulin "stress" hormone)
  Oral contraceptives (causes insulin resistance)
  Thiazides (causes insulin resistance)

Furosemide

- Iatrogenic etiologies (excessive rates of parenteral glucose infusion)
  Intravenous glucose infusion
  Hyperalimentation
- Acute pancreatitis (transient pancreatic islet ß-cell dysfunction)
- Head injury (dysfunctional autonomic control of the pancreatic islets)

Diabetes mellitus is the family of metabolic diseases characterized by sustained (chronic) hyperglycemia. In some cases, prolonged use of a medication such as glucocorticoids causes diabetes mellitus. However, discontinuation of the medication should lead to a reversal of the diabetic state.

Diabetes mellitus results from a decline in insulin action. Insulin action is the approximate multiplicative product of the absolute insulin concentration and the insulin sensitivity of the tissues. The three major targets for insulin action are the liver, muscle, and adipose tissue. In the liver, insulin stimulates glycolysis sparing free fatty acids for triglyceride synthesis. Gluconeogenesis is also suppressed making amino acids available for protein synthesis. Insulin promotes energy storage through stimulation of glycogen synthesis. The net effect of insulin on the liver is increased glucose utilization and decreased hepatic glucose output (HGO).

In muscle and adipose tissue, insulin stimulates the migration of insulin-responsive glucose transporters (GLUT4) to the cell membrane permitting increased rates of glucose uptake by these tissues. Adipose tissue burns glucose to acetate (e.g., acetyl-CoA) that is substrate for fatty acid synthesis and subsequent triglyceride synthesis. While burning glucose for energy, muscle will also store glucose as muscle glycogen. All three tissues increase glucose clearance from the circulation with a resultant fall in plasma glucose concentrations.

X) Clinical Symptoms Of Diabetes Mellitus

When the plasma glucose level exceeds the renal threshold for glucose (e.g., more glucose is filtered by the glomerulus than can be reabsorbed by the renal tubules), glycosuria results. Because of the resulting elevated urine osmolality, a diuresis ensues that is clinically evident as polyuria (increased urination). Patients will frequently begin to void at night (nocturia) while children may experience enuresis (bed wetting). With increased urinary fluid loss, thirst is stimulated causing polydipsia (increased drinking). Because of diminished insulin action, adipose tissue lipolysis increases. As well, protein catabolism accelerates to provide amino acid carbon skeletons for gluconeogenesis in the liver. The clinical consequence of this catabolic state is weight loss. Some patients experience increased appetite (e.g., polyphagia). Blurred vision may occur resulting from fluid shifts involving the lens of the eye secondary to hyperglycemia. Children who are in very poor diabetic control may grow poorly. However, poor growth in diabetic children is the exception and not the rule. Hyperglycemia clearly impairs phagocyte function. When impaired native (e.g., intrinsic or natural immunity) immunity is combined with the "nutrient-rich" tissue and body fluid conditions provided by hyperglycemia, increased susceptibility to bacterial infection often occurs. Diabetic subjects are predisposed to soft-tissue bacterial infections, balanitis (infection of the space between the foreskin and glans), vaginitis, and urinary tract infections. Severe acute insulin deficiency can precipitate diabetic ketoacidosis (DKA). DKA is fatal in 10-15% of adults and 0.5% of children that experience this condition.

For patients who have had diabetes 10 or more years, there is an increasing likelihood that they will experience diabetic complications. These problems include macrovascular, microvascular, and neuropathic diseases. Macrovascular disease may present as angina, heart attack (myocardial infarction), or heart failure (chronic coronary artery disease), stroke (cerebrovascular disease), or claudication (peripheral vascular disease). Claudication is the pain and fatigue that patients experience in their legs when walking when there is inadequate blood supply to match oxygen demand. Microvascular disease produces retinopathy and nephropathy. Retinopathy can lead to blindness while nephropathy can lead to renal failure. Peripheral neuropathy can produce loss of sensation in the feet and hands. Painful peripheral neuropathy can be incapacitating. Autonomic neuropathy may be evidenced in gastroparesis (decreased gastrointestinal tract motility), impotence, decreased sexual response in women, postural hypotension (low blood pressure upon arising from the sitting or supine position often accompanied by light-headedness or fainting), and loss of the normal beat-to-beat variation in heart rate that occurs with breathing.

XI) Classification Of Diabetes Mellitus

Chronic (sustained) hyperglycemia may be permanent (e.g., type 1 or type 2 diabetes mellitus) or time-limited [e.g., gestational diabetes mellitus (diabetes during pregnancy that resolves following delivery]. Diabetes is now classified into 4 subtypes:

1) Type 1 diabetes mellitus
2) Type 2 diabetes mellitus
3) Other specific types of diabetes mellitus
4) Gestational diabetes mellitus (GDM)

The classification of diabetes mellitus is based upon etiology and not the type of therapy that a patient receives. The terms "previous abnormality of glucose tolerance" and "potential abnormality of glucose tolerance" are no longer used. Likewise, the nomenclature "insulin-dependent diabetes mellitus (IDDM)," "type I (Roman numeral) diabetes mellitus," "non-insulin-dependent diabetes mellitus (NIDDM)," and "type II (Roman numeral) diabetes mellitus" is replaced by the terms type 1 (Arabic) and type 2 (Arabic) diabetes mellitus.

Type 1 diabetes mellitus results from absolute insulinopenia (low insulin concentration in the blood stream). Insulinopenia most commonly results from autoimmune destruction of the insulin-producing beta cells. This condition is frequently accompanied by the expression of several islet autoantibodies that can be recognized at or before the time of diagnosis of type 1 diabetes mellitus. The presence of islet cell autoantibodies (ICA, detected by indirect immunofluorescence), insulin autoantibodies (IAA), glutamic acid decarboxylase autoantibodies (GADA), IA-2 or IA-2ß autoantibodies (islet tyrosine phosphatases; IAA, GADA, IA-2A, IA-2ßA are detected by radioimmunoprecipitation techniques) indicate an autoimmune etiology for diabetes mellitus and classification as "type 1" diabetes mellitus. Indeed, if the clinical differentiation between type 1 and type 2 diabetes mellitus is problematic in a patient, measurement of islet autoantibodies should strongly be considered. When the cause of the insulinopenia is unidentified, diabetes mellitus is also classified as "type 1" diabetes mellitus. If a specific non-autoimmune etiology for the insulinopenia is identified [e.g., beta-cell destruction from Vacor (rat poison)], the diabetes mellitus is then classified under the heading of "other specific types of diabetes mellitus" (see below).

Type 2 diabetes mellitus results from a combination of tissue insulin resistance and relative beta cell failure (e.g., relative insulinopenia). Relative insulinopenia infers that even if the absolute concentration of insulin in the circulation is greater than normal, the supra-normal insulin concentration is still *insufficient* to correct the patient's hyperglycemia. Insulin resistance is most often post-receptor, e.g., the insulin receptor is structurally normal; however, there is deficient generation of second messengers within the target cell leading to decreased insulin action.

Once the pathogenesis of an initially "idiopathic" form of type 1 or type 2 diabetes mellitus is discovered, the diabetes mellitus is reassigned as "other specific type." Other specific types are subclassified into eight subtypes:

1) Genetic defects of ß-cell function

2) Genetic defects in insulin action

3) Diseases of the exocrine pancreas

4) Endocrinopathies

5) Drug- or chemical-induced diabetes

6) Infections

7) Uncommon forms of immune-mediated diabetes

8) Other genetic syndromes associated with diabetes

ß-cell dysfunction can result from mutations in hepatic nuclear factors 4α (HNF-4α), 1α (HNF-1α) or glucokinase producing maturity-onset diabetes of the young (MODY). MODY is a form of type 2 diabetes mellitus that presents before age 25 that is inherited as an autosomal dominant trait. Mitochondrial mutations (e.g., A3243G) have been associated with diabetes mellitus and deafness. Mitochondrial diseases are inherited strictly from the mother as the conceptus' mitochondria are provided by the ovum and not the sperm. Insulinopathies [missense mutations in insulin especially at amino acids 25 or 26 in the beta chain (both normally phenylalanine) and in amino acid 3 in the alpha chain (normally valine)] and hyperproinsulinopathies (e.g., incomplete cleavage of proinsulin into insulin and C-peptide) are rare causes of diabetes mellitus.

Many insulin receptor mutations have been described that involve the alpha or beta chains. However, these mutations are rare in the general population of patients with type 2 diabetes mellitus. The most common diseases of the exocrine pancreas to produce diabetes are cystic fibrosis and chronic pancreatitis. Numerous endocrinopathies cause diabetes mellitus including Cushing syndrome, acromegaly (growth hormone excess), and pheochromocytoma. Chronic use of glucocorticoids, growth hormone, or catecholamines can lead to diabetes mellitus. Diabetes secondary to pentamidine has been observed in AIDS patients who have been treated for *Pneumocystis carinii* pneumonia. In such cases, pentamidine causes beta-cell necrosis. The rat poison Vacor[R] has caused diabetes mellitus. Through their effects on the anti-insulin hormones, infection may produce a diabetic state; however, this state usually remits with resolution of the infection.

Uncommon forms of immune-mediated diabetes include anti-insulin receptor autoantibodies that can produce profound insulin resistance. While autoimmune hypoglycemia from anti-insulin autoantibodies is best well known for its hypoglycemic symptoms, glucose intolerance can also be observed in this rare autoimmune condition.

Many genetic syndromes are associated with diabetes mellitus such as lipodystrophy (abnormal fat distribution), Werner syndrome, and myotonic dystrophy.

Gestational diabetes mellitus (GDM) is diabetes mellitus that develops during pregnancy. In the ADA guidelines, GDM includes "any degree of glucose intolerance with onset or first recognition during pregnancy." GDM usually remits following delivery; however, women with GDM are at increased risk of developing type 2 diabetes mellitus later in life. There are serious adverse fetal health consequences when maternal diabetes mellitus is unrecognized. These complications include macrosomia (large size) that can lead to difficult delivery (e.g, "dystocia"), and hypoglycemia or hypocalcemia in the immediate newborn period. Infants born to diabetic mothers (IDM) are also at higher risk for respiratory distress syndrome and hyperbilirubinemia than age-matched infants.

XII) Diagnosis Of Diabetes Mellitus

The preferred specimen for the diagnosis of diabetes mellitus is a fasting plasma glucose determination. Patients should fast overnight at least 8 hours but not longer than 16 hours. Other than water, patients must not eat, smoke, or take medications until the sample is drawn. Excluding acutely ill patients with obvious signs and symptoms of diabetes mellitus and unquestionable hyperglycemia (e.g., plasma glucose levels >300-400 mg/dL), acute illness or hospitalization within the previous 6 to 8 weeks are relative contraindications to testing because severe acute illness can cause transient hyperglycemia. As well, patients recovering from surgery, especially intra-abdominal surgery, may be poorly nourished and may be glucose intolerant because of inadequate caloric intake.

Unless the blood specimen is rapidly analyzed (e.g., the plasma is separated from the cells in ≤60 minutes, or the chemical analysis is performed in ≤60 minutes), sodium fluoride (NaF) containing "gray-top" tubes should be used (10-30 mg per 5 mL of whole blood). NaF poisons glycolysis inhibiting the usually observed 5-7%/hour fall in serum glucose that results from white blood cell metabolism of glucose. NaF is also a weak anticoagulant. However if blood is allowed to stand for more than a few hours (e.g., ≥2-4 hours), oxalate ($K_2C_2O_4$; 2 mg/mL whole blood) should also be added to the NaF tube to insure anticoagulation (e.g., plasma and not serum). A partially anticoagulated sample is technically highly undesirable because fibrin clots commonly obstruct instrumentation pipettes, ports, and tubing.

If the fasting plasma glucose is <126 mg/dL and diabetes is a serious clinical consideration, an oral glucose tolerance test (OGTT) should be performed. The 1997 ADA guidelines simplify the OGTT to a fasting sample and 2 hour plasma glucose measurement. The only exception to the "2-2 OGTT" (2 samples-2 hours) is OGTT testing during pregnancy as will be described below. Similar to isolated fasting plasma glucose determinations, preanalytic considerations are important: a regular diet of ≥100-150 gm of carbohydrate per day for at least 3 days prior to testing, no acute severe illnesses (an upper respiratory tract infection is not a contraindication to testing, however the "flu" with vomiting and diarrhea would be a contraindication), no recent hospitalizations, and unrestricted activity prior to testing is necessary. Outside of pregnancy where 100 gm of glucose is administered, adults receive 75 gm of anhydrous glucose dissolved in a favored drink (e.g., Glucola). In children, 1.75 gm/kg of glucose is administered to a maximum dose of 75 gm. Time zero is when the patient begins to ingest the glucose load and the beverage should be consumed in ≤5 minutes. In the drink, the maximum glucose concentration is 25 gm/dL.

The diagnostic criteria presented below are those recommended by the ADA as published in the July 1997 issue of *Diabetes Care*. These criteria apply equally to children and adults. This is an important change in diagnostic criteria because the 1979 National Diabetes Data Group (NDDG) recommendations had somewhat different OGTT cutoffs for adults and children.

At least one of the following three criteria must be met on two occasions in order to establish the diagnosis of diabetes:

1) Symptoms of diabetes mellitus plus any random plasma glucose measurement ≥200 mg/dL (≥11.1 mmol/L);
2) Fasting plasma glucose ≥126 mg/dL (≥7 mmol/L);
3) During an OGTT, the 2 hour plasma glucose ≥200 mg/dL (≥11.1 mmol/L).

Unless severe symptoms (e.g., unquestionable polyuria, polydipsia, weight loss or diabetic ketoacidosis) and profound hyperglycemia (e.g., plasma glucose >300-400 mg/dL) are present, *the initial findings must be confirmed on a subsequent occasion.* There is no specific guideline as to how soon the "confirmatory" test should be performed. Also, the first and second test need *not* be the same test. If an OGTT has been planned and the fasting plasma glucose is ≥126 mg/dL, there is no reason to administer the oral glucose load or measure a 2 hour specimen. As noted above, IFG is present when the fasting plasma glucose is between 110 mg/dL and 125 mg/dL. Impaired glucose tolerance (IGT) is defined as a 2 hour plasma glucose level of 140 mg/dL to 199 mg/dL. IFG and IGT predict a markedly increased risk of developing type 2 diabetes mellitus in the future.

Because of the adverse effects of diabetes on the fetus, the American College of Obstetrics and Gynecology (ACOG) recommends that all women undergo diabetes screening by 24 to 28 weeks gestation. The ADA also recommends screening for GDM unless the pregnant woman is considered to be at low risk for GDM.

"Low risk" is defined by the ADA as: 1) maternal age <25 years, 2) normal body weight, 3) lack of family history of diabetes, and 4) ethnicity other than African American, Hispanic American, or Native American. The screening OGTT consists of a 50 gm glucose load with measurement of a 1 hour post-load plasma glucose. The patient need not be fasting. If this value is ≥140 mg/dL, a diagnostic 3 hour OGTT is performed with a 100 gm glucose load. For the 3 hour OGTT, 4 time points are assessed: fasting, 1 hour, 2 hours, and 3 hours. If the initial fasting plasma glucose is ≥126 mg/dL, diabetes is present and the test can be terminated. GDM is diagnosed when any 2 values are met or exceeded:

- Fasting 105 mg/dL
- 1 hour 190 mg/dL
- 2 hours 165 mg/dL
- 3 hours 145 mg/dL

Analytically, plasma and serum glucose levels are essentially identical. Whole blood glucose values are ~20 mg/dL lower than plasma or serum because whole blood contains solid elements (e.g., the non-aqueous portion of red blood cells). In the fasting state, capillary and whole blood venous glucose values are equivalent. However following a glucose load, capillary values are ~20 mg/dL higher than whole blood venous values.

XIII) Screening Strategies For Diabetes Mellitus

In the new 1997 ADA recommendations, all nondiabetic adults over age 45 should have a measurement of fasting plasma glucose every 3 years. This is because the frequency of diabetes mellitus rises sixfold between ages 40 and 45. Furthermore, many type 2 diabetes mellitus patients already have complications at the time of clinical diagnosis. This indicates that by awaiting the *clinical* presentation of type 2 diabetes (e.g., polyuria, polydipsia, etc.) or a fasting plasma glucose value ≥140 mg/dL (the old cutoff), the *biochemical* diagnosis of type 2 diabetes is significantly delayed and thus biochemical screening is warranted using the revised diabetes cutoff of ≥126 mg/dL.

Screening for diabetes mellitus should be carried out *before age 45* when: 1) obesity is present, 2) there is a family history of diabetes in a first degree relative, 3) the individual is a member of a high-risk group for diabetes mellitus (e.g., African, Hispanic, or Native American), 4) there is a history of GDM or delivering a baby >9 lb, 4) the patient is hypertensive (≥140/90), 5) the HDL cholesterol level is low (e.g., ≤35 mg/dL), 6) the triglyceride levels are elevated (e.g., ≥250 mg/dL), or 7) there is a history of previous IFG or IGT. Screening in pregnancy was discussed previously.

XIV) Biochemical Monitoring In Diabetes Mellitus

The goal of therapy in caring for individuals with diabetes is: 1) elimination of symptoms, 2) control of the PG, lipids, blood pressure, etc. to delay or prevent diabetic complications. In children with diabetes, a further goal of diabetes care is to insure normal growth and development. Routine laboratory assessments are vital to the monitoring of diabetes in optimizing clinical management. These assessments fall into four major categories: 1) Self-blood glucose monitoring (SBGM), 2) Long term assessment of diabetic control, 3) Evaluation of lipid status, and 4) Renal evaluation.

Self-blood glucose monitoring

SBGM is the cornerstone of daily diabetes management for the patient afflicted with diabetes. With SBGM, the patient can measure his or her capillary glucose any time of the day or night as needed to make informed choices about diet, exercise, and insulin administration. In insulin treated patients, SBGM should be performed 3 to 4 times per day and more often as required. Treatment algorithms can assist in making informed changes in insulin dosing. SBGM systems measure capillary glucose by applying whole blood to reagent-embedded strips. After a chemical reaction occurs in the strip, glucose induces a color change proportionate the capillary glucose concentration. The strips in some cases can be read visually; however, all systems on the market today are designed to be read by meters that provide more accurate measurements than visual interpretations. By necessity, patients must use a microlancet to draw a drop of blood from the finger for self monitoring. Meters for SBGM display coefficients of variation of 2 to 5% when used by well trained individuals. However in practice, up to half of all results vary >20% from values obtained in a central laboratory. This points out the need for proper training, instrument maintenance, control sample testing, and yearly validation of the monitor's performance compared with the central laboratory.

Assessment of diabetic control

Until the development of assays for glycosylated hemoglobin, there was no way to objectively assess the patient's long term glycemic control. Glycosylated hemoglobin results from the nonenzymatic addition of glucose to the hemoglobin molecules inside red blood cells. Biochemically, glucose first forms a reversible (labile) product with amine groups of hemoglobin forming an aldimine (Schiff base). A nonreversible Amadori rearrangement then occurs to form a ketoamine. Since the average red blood cell life span is 120 days, glycohemoglobin measurements represent the mean PG of the previous 2 to 3 months. Therefore, glycohemoglobin concentration is proportional to the elevation and duration of elevation of the PG level. Glycohemoglobin is not one molecule. Glycohemoglobin includes three forms of glycosylated hemoglobin A: hemoglobin A_{1a}, hemoglobin A_{1b}, and hemoglobin A_{1c}. Hemoglobin A_{1a} is composed of two subfractions: A_{1a1} (fructose-1,6-diphosphate bound to the beta chain) and A_{1a2} (glucose-6-phosphate bound to the beta chain). The structure of hemoglobin A_{1b} is unknown. In hemoglobin A_{1c}, the N-terminal valine of the ß-chain is glycosylated. On average, hemoglobin A_{1c} represents ~75-80% of glycosylated hemoglobin. Total glycohemoglobin or hemoglobin A_{1c} are expressed as a percent of the total hemoglobin (hemoglobin A_o plus glycohemoglobin) where hemoglobin A_o is non-glycosylated hemoglobin A.

Clinical situations where red blood cell survival is shortened will falsely depress glycohemoglobin measurements. Such situations include hemolysis, hereditary spherocytosis, and hypersplenism. Likewise, prolonged red blood cell survival as seen with polycythemia or following splenectomy can falsely raise glycohemoglobin concentrations.

Glycosylated hemoglobin species can be measured by a wide variety of techniques including ion exchange or affinity column chromatography, electrophoresis, ion exchange high performance liquid chromatography (HPLC), and immunoassay. A glycohemoglobin assay should be chosen that is traceable to the DCCT reference method (HPLC). Assay certification for manufacturers is supplied by the National Glycohemoglobin Standardization Program.

The ADA recommends that glycohemoglobin be monitored at the time of initial clinical assessment to document the degree of glycemic control and regularly thereafter. Unless the patient is in excellent control (hemoglobin A1c <7%) when glycohemoglobin can be measured as infrequently as every 6 months, monitoring glycohemoglobin every 3 months is appropriate.

In pregnant patients and in patients with certain hemoglobinopathies (e.g., SS, SC, or CC) where there is no hemoglobin A_0 to be glycosylated, glycated serum proteins can be monitored. Total glycated serum protein, or more often measured, glycated albumin reflects ~10 days of glycemic control. The glycated albumin assay detects fructosamine and thus "fructosamine" is the test often ordered for measurement of glycated albumin. Because this test only displays short term control, other than the clinical conditions outlined above, glycohemoglobin measurements are preferred over glycated albumin measurements.

Evaluation of lipid status

Macrovascular disease is a leading cause of death in both type 1 diabetes and type 2 diabetes. Therefore, lipid profile measurements (total cholesterol, triglycerides, HDL cholesterol, and calculated LDL cholesterol) play a major role in the routine laboratory evaluation of patients with diabetes. Adults with diabetes should have a yearly lipid profile measured. Risk assessment is depicted below:

	DESIRABLE	BORDERLINE	UNDESIRABLE
LDL cholesterol	<100	100-129	≥130
Triglycerides	<200	200-399	≥400
HDL cholesterol	>45	35-45	<35

Note that these adult LDL cholesterol guidelines for patients with diabetes are more stringent than the routine guidelines provided by the National Cholesterol Education Program for nondiabetic adults.

In children, lipids are measured at the time of diagnosis and after glycemic control is established. If the values fall within the desirable range, according to the ADA guidelines, lipids need not be repeated for another 5 years. Otherwise, the NCEP guidelines for children are recommended. However it is the author's opinion that a yearly lipid profile should be obtained in all diabetic children similar to adults. This is because triglyceride measurements are a monitor of diabetic control and therapy (in the authors opinion) for elevated LDL cholesterol levels should be very aggressive because of the high morbidity and mortality of macrovascular disease in patients with type 1 diabetes. We would predict that earlier treatment of hypercholesterolemia would be more effective in preventing atherosclerosis. See chapter 7 for a further discussion of lipids.

Renal evaluation

In adults, a yearly urinalysis is recommended by the ADA. If this dipstick test for protein is negative, microalbuminuria should be sought. In adults, testing for microalbuminuria should be performed at the time of diagnosis and yearly thereafter. After 5 years of diabetes in children, microalbuminuria should be sought and yearly thereafter assuming the dipstick is negative for protein. Microalbuminuria can be measured in a 24 hour collection, in a timed collection less than 24 hours, and in a spot sample. In all situations, urinary creatinine is measured. In the timed collections, urinary creatinine permits an assessment of the completeness of collection. For spot samples, the albumin to creatinine ratio is calculated. While cutoffs are laboratory specific, general interpretative guidelines are outlined below:

	NORMAL	MICROALBUMINURIA	CLINICAL ALBUMINURIA
Spot urine (µg/mg creatinine)	<30	30-300	>300
Timed sample (µg/min)	<20	20-200	>200
24 hr sample (mg/24 hr)	<30	30-300	>300

If the dipstick is positive for protein, the clinician should order a 24 hour urine collection and serum creatinine measurement for determination 24 hour protein excretion and calculation of the creatinine clearance.

Urine glucose testing is discouraged and has been replaced by SBGM. When patients are ill or moderately to markedly hyperglycemic (e.g., PG ≥240-300 mg/dL), urine ketones should be measured.

XV) Summary

Diabetes mellitus is a state of chronic hyperglycemia with many adverse consequences for the individual and society. Good diabetes control decreases the risk of microvascular complications in type 1 diabetes mellitus. Earlier diagnosis and better control of hyperglycemia are also likely to delay or prevent the complications of type 2 diabetes mellitus. The frequency of type 2 diabetes mellitus in the general population is rising and is most likely due to the high frequency of obesity now observed in the general population.

The 1997 ADA guidelines greatly simplify the diagnosis of diabetes mellitus. The cutoff for fasting hyperglycemia is now 126 mg/dL. Excluding pregnancy, the OGTT is simplified to 2 samples: fasting and 2 hours. The ≥126 mg/dL fasting plasma glucose cutoff and the 2 hour OGTT cutoff of ≥200 mg/dL identify similar populations of hyperglycemic (diabetic) individuals.

Screening for diabetes mellitus should be carried out under rigorous, controlled conditions to insure accurate diagnosis. Presently, glycated hemoglobin determinations (e.g., hemoglobin A_{1c}) are useful for following the clinical course of patients diagnosed with diabetes. However, glycated hemoglobin measurements should not be used to screen for diabetes. For example, glycated hemoglobin levels within the reference range do not exclude the diagnosis of diabetes mellitus when the hyperglycemia is of acute onset or of only short duration (e.g., in type 1 diabetes mellitus or very early type 2 diabetes mellitus). Assay standardization and re-evaluation of reference ranges (e.g., clear exclusion of individuals with either IFG or IGT) may permit glycated hemoglobin measurements to someday play a role in diabetes screening.

For patients with established diabetes who are dipstick protein negative, yearly microalbumin determinations can detect incipient nephropathy. Likewise, lipid monitoring and treatment is very important for the prevention of macrovascular complications.

References

1) Raskin P: "Reactive hypoglycemia"-a clinical unicorn. Clin Diabetes 1985;3(4):74.

2) Parardy J, Havrankova J, Lepage R, et al. Blood glucose measurements during symptomatic episodes in patients with suspected postprandial hypoglycemia. N Eng J Med 1989;321:1421-5.

3) Finegold DN, Stanley CA, Baker L. Glycemic response to glucagon during fasting: an aid in the diagnosis of hyperinsulinism. J Pediatrics 1980;96:257-9.

4) Lebowitz MR, Blumenthal SA. The molar ratio of insulin to C-peptide. Arch Intern Med 1993;153:650-5.

5) Service FJ, O'Brien PC, McMahon MM, Kao PC. C-peptide during prolonged fast in insulinoma. J Clin Endo Metab 1993;76:655-9.

6) Daughaday WH, Emanuele MA, Brooks MH, Brabato AL, Kapadia M, Rotwein P. Synthesis and secretion of insulin-like growth factor II by a leiomyosarcoma with associated hypoglycemia. N Engl J Med 1988;319:1434-40.

7) Winter, W.E. Laboratory Approaches to Thyroid and Adrenal Function Testing: . American Association for Clinical Chemistry, Inc., (Monograph), Washington D.C., 1995: in press.

General references concerning Hypoglycemia

1) Service FJ: Clinical Review 42: Hypoglycemias. J Clin Endo Metab 1993;76:269-72.

2) Winter, W.E. Diabetes Mellitus: Pathophysiology, Etiologies, Complications, Management, and Laboratory Evaluation. American Association for Clinical Chemistry, Inc., (Monograph), Washington D.C., 1994: 1-84.

3) O'Brien T, O'Brien PC, Service FJ. Insulin surrogates in insulinoma. J Clin Endo Metab 1993;77:448-51.

4) Chaussain J-L, Goegres P, Gendrel D, Donnadieu, Job J-C. Serum branched-chain amino acids in the diagnosis of hyperinsulinism in infancy. J Pediatrics 1980; 96:923-6.

5) Winter, W.E.: Laboratory approaches to the evaluation of hypoglycemia. AACC Endocrine/Toxicology In-Service Training and Continuing Education 1995; 13(5):139-150.

General references concerning Hyperglycemia

1) Diabetes Mellitus: Pathophysiology, Etiologies, Complications, Management, and Laboratory Evaluation, Winter, W.E.: American Association for Clinical Chemistry, Inc., (Monograph), Washington D.C., 1994; 1-84

2) Expert Committee: Report of the expert committee on the diagnosis and classification of diabetes mellitus. Diabetes Care 1997; 20:1183-97

3) National Diabetes Data Group: Classification and diagnosis of diabetes mellitus and other categories of glucose intolerance. Diabetes 1979; 28:1039-1057

4) Wilkin's-The Diagnosis and Treatment of Endocrine Disorders in Childhood and Adolescence, 4th edition, Winter, W.E.: Autoimmune Endocrinopathies. In: M.S. Kappy R.M. Blizzard, C.J. Migeon,(eds): Charles C. Thomas Co. Publishers Springfield, IL; February, 1994; 317-382.

7
Laboratory Diagnosis of Lipoprotein Disorders

I. JIALAL, MD, PHD, FRCPATH, DABCC

A.) Background

Disturbances in lipoprotein metabolism have two major clinical sequelae in man. Hypercholesterolemia and/or low levels of HDL-cholesterol can predispose to premature atherosclerosis while very high levels of plasma triglyceride (greater than 1000 mg/dL) can predispose to pancreatitis. Two of the major lipid components in plasma are cholesterol and triglyceride. However, both cholesterol and triglyceride are insoluble in water and in order to be transported to the various tissues they must be packaged into a lipoprotein particle, the core of which comprises the cholesteryl esters and triglycerides and the surface which comprises phospholipids, apolipoproteins, and free cholesterol. This lipoprotein particle is now water soluble and can be transported in plasma. In man, there are four major lipoprotein classes, as shown in Table I, and they can be classified either by their density or electrophoretic mobility. Chylomicrons and very low density lipoprotein (VLDL) are mainly triglyceride carrying particles. Low density lipoproteins (LDL) and high density lipoproteins (HDL) are the major cholesterol carrying particles. It is important to note, from Table I, that all the major lipoprotein classes comprise cholesterol, triglycerides, phospholipid and apolipoprotein and the concentrations of these various moieties are different in the various lipoprotein classes. Dietary fat is packaged in the intestine as a chylomicron particle, which is then secreted into the plasma via the thoracic duct. In the plasma, chylomicrons are acted upon by a pivotal enzyme in lipoprotein metabolism, lipoprotein lipase (LPL), which requires apolipoprotein C-II as its co-factor. Following the action of LPL, the chylomicron remnants are then taken up and metabolized further by the liver. VLDL, which comprises mainly triglyceride, is secreted by the liver, and on entry into the circulation it has the same fate as chylomicrons in that it is acted on by LPL to result in the formation of remnants such as intermediate density lipoprotein (IDL). The IDL can then be processed by the liver or can continue to lose triglycerides further and comprise a particle that is essentially cholesterol and apolipoprotein B-100. This is low density lipoprotein (LDL). LDL is then processed by the low density lipoprotein receptor, which was elegantly elucidated by Goldstein and Brown. Finally, while we do not understand the precise mechanism by which high density lipoprotein functions, it is generally believed that it participates in reverse cholesterol transport in that HDL picks up the unesterified cholesterol, esterifies the cholesterol via the en-

TABLE I. COMPOSITION AND PROPERTIES OF MAJOR LIPOPROTEINS

	CHYLOMICRONS	VLDL	LDL	HDL
Origin	Gut	Liver	VLDL and IDL	Liver, gut, intravascular metabolism
Density (g ml^{-1})	0.94	0.94-1.006	1.019 1.063	1.063-1.21
Electrophorectic mobility	Origin	Pre-beta	Beta	Alpha
Major apoproteins	B-48, C, E	B-100, C, E	B-100	A-I, A-II, C, E
Protein (%)	1%	10%	20%	50%
Major lipid (%)	Triglyceride (90%)	Triglyceride (55%)	Cholesterol (50%)	Phospholipid (25%) Cholesterol (20%)
Function	Transport dietary triglycerides mainly	Transport endogenous triglycerides mainly	Transport of cholesterol esters	Reverse cholesterol transport

zyme lecithin cholesterol acyltransferase and then shuttles the cholesterol back to the liver for excretion as bile acids and neutral sterols. Since HDL contains the antioxidants, paraoxonase and platelet activating factor acetyl hydrolase, it is an important reservoir for antioxidants.

B.) Dyslipidemia

A practical classification of the major forms of dyslipidemia includes hypercholesterolemia, hypertriglyceridemia, combined hyperlipidemias, and low levels of HDL-cholesterol. A lipoprotein disorder can either be primary or secondary. There are several classifications of lipoprotein disorders, none of which are entirely satisfactory. The classification of the familial hyperlipoproteinemias are shown in Table II. The most practical approach to the hyperlipoproteinemia would be to look at the lipoproteins that are abnormal and pursue their investigation. Thus, in this chapter, for the sake of simplicity, the hyperlipidemias will be discussed under the following headings: Hypercholesterolemia, Low Levels of HDL Cholesterol, Hypertriglyceridemia, and Combined Hyperlipidemia.

1.) Hypercholesterolemia

The classification of hypercholesterolemia, was recently reported by the National Cholesterol Education Program's Adult Treatment Panel II (ATP II). In adults an elevated serum cholesterol is defined as a value ≥240 mg/dL; a borderline cholesterol is between 200-239 mg/dL and a desirable serum cholesterol is below 200 mg/dL. Also included now in the initial classification is the HDL cholesterol. An HDL cholesterol level below 35 mg/dL is defined as low and constitutes an independent coronary artery disease (CAD) risk factor. In children, elevated cholesterol is ≥ 200mg/dL, borderline 170-199 mg/dL and desirable < 170mg/dL. Since both the total cholesterol and HDL cholesterol can be obtained on a non-fasting sample, a lipoprotein analysis to determine the LDL cholesterol is reserved for patients with an elevated total cholesterol (≥240 mg/dL), a borderline high blood cholesterol (200-239 mg/dL), with an HDL cholesterol below 35 mg/dL or two or more coronary risk factors, as shown in Table 3. It should be pointed out that HDL cholesterol ≥60 mg/dL is now considered beneficial and thus 1 risk factor is subtracted in the borderline group. Previously, a desirable blood cholesterol below 200 mg/dL was considered normal. Now according to the recent guidelines of the ATP, if these subjects have an HDL cholesterol below 35 mg/dL, they also should have a lipoprotein analysis to determined the LDL cholesterol to decide on further management. Desirable LDL cholesterol in adults is <130

TABLE 2. FAMILIAL HYPERLIPOPROTEINEMIAS

GENETIC DISORDER	PHENOTYPE	BIOCHEMICAL DEFECT	CLINICAL PRESENTATION	CHOLESTEROL	TRIGLYCERIDES
Familial LPL deficiency	I	Absence of LPL activity	Eruptive xanthoma; hepatosplenomegaly, pancreatitis	increased +	increased +++
Familial apo C-II deficiency	I or V	Absence or abnormal structure of apo C-II	Pancreatitis	increased +	increased +++
Familial hypercholesterolemia	IIa or IIb	Deficiency of LDL receptors	Tendinous and tuberous xanthoma; premature atherosclerosis	increased +++	N(a) or increased + (IIb)
Familial dysbetalipoproteinemia	III	Abnormal apo E and defect in triglyceride-rich lipoprotein metabolism	Tubero-eruptive and planar xanthoma; premature atherosclerosis	increased ++	increased ++
Familial combined hyperlipidemia	IIa, IIb or IV	Unknown	Premature atherosclerosis	increased or N	increased or N
Familial hypertriglyceridemias	IV and V	Unknown	Type V: Eruptive xanthoma; hepatosplenomegaly; pancreatitis	N (IV) increased + (V)	increased + (IV) increased +++ (V)

N = normal

mg/dL, borderline elevated is 130-160, and elevated is >160 mg/dL. Desirable LDL cholesterol in children is <110 mg/dL, borderline elevated is 110-129 mg/dL, and elevated is ≥130 mg/dL.

Having established that a patient has a hypercholesterolemia with an elevated level of LDL cholesterol, it is important to exclude a secondary cause of hypercholesterolemia. Some of the more common causes of hypercholesterolemia that need to be ruled out in these patients are shown in Table 4. The classical single gene disorder that results in hypercholesterolemia is familial hypercholesterolemia. This is an autosomal dominant disorder characterized by increased levels of LDL cholesterol due to a genetic defect resulting in decreased activity of LDL receptors. Familial hypercholesterolemia (FH) can present in either the homozygous or the heterozygous state. The homozygote presents in pediatric practice and these children have few or no LDL receptors resulting in marked elevations in LDL cholesterol, xanthoma formation on the skin and tendons and premature atherosclerosis. The more common variety, which presents in adults, is the heterozygote in whom there is about a 50% reduction in LDL receptors resulting in a twofold increase in LDL cholesterol. They also could present with tendon xanthoma and premature atherosclerosis manifesting in early to middle adulthood. To date, numerous mutations of the LDL receptor gene have been described. Familial hypercholesterolemia can be sub-classified into two types, depending on the plasma triglyceride. In the Type II-A disorder, the plasma triglycerides are normal, while in the Type II-B disorder, plasma triglycerides are also increased.

TABLE 3. CAD RISK FACTORS

Positive

Age,

- Men ≥ 45 years
- Women ≥ 55 or premature menopause without estrogen replacement therapy

Family history of premature coronary heart disease

Smoking

Hypertension

HDL Cholesterol < 35 mg/dL (0.9 mmol/L)

Diabetes

Negative

- HDL Cholesterol ≥ 60 mg/dL (1.6 mmol/L)

Adapted from Adult Panel II. JAMA 1993;269:3015-3023.

Familial hypercholesterolemia is not the most common cause of the Type II-A phenotype. Primary moderate hypercholesterolemia is the most common cause for an isolated increase in LDL cholesterol. This is believed to be due to a complex interaction of genetic and environmental factors and has been referred to as polygenic hypercholesterolemia. Recently a mutation in the receptor binding region of apoprotein B-100 at position 3500 has been shown to result in a defective apo-B that interferes with binding to the LDL receptor resulting in an elevated LDL cholesterol. This type of dyslipidemia has been named familial defective apolipoprotein B.

Unlike in adults, universal pediatric cholesterol screening is not recommended. A strategy was developed by the NCEP Expert Panel on blood cholesterol levels in children and adolescents to identify those most likely to be at increased risk for developing premature coronary artery disease. Recommendations were made based on a family history of coronary artery disease, hypercholesterolemia, or if they had two or more risk factors. It is recommended that a lipoprotein profile be performed in children and adolescents whose parents or grandparents at age 55 years or younger underwent coronary angiography and were found to have coronary atherosclerosis, in children and adolescents whose parents or grand-

TABLE 4. CAUSES OF SECONDARY HYPERLIPIDEMIA

1. PREDOMINANTLY HYPERTRIGLYCERIDEMIA
Obesity
Diabetes Mellitus
Alcoholism
Renal failure
Lipodystrophy
Dysglobulinemias
Estrogen therapy
Steroid therapy
Beta blocker therapy
Isotretinoin therapy
2. PREDOMINANTLY HYPERCHOLESTEROLEMIA
Hypothyroidism
Cholestasis
Nephrotic syndrome
Dysglobulinemias
Diuretics
Cyclosporin

parents at age 55 years or less had suffered a previously documented myocardial infarction, angina pectoris, peripheral vascular disease, cerebrovascular disease, or sudden cardiac death. Screening for hypercholesterolemia should be undertaken in the offspring of a parent who has been found to have a high blood cholesterol (≥240 mg/dL) and when the parent or grandparental history is unavailable with children and adolescents who have two or more cardiovascular risk factors. It is recommended that at least a total cholesterol level should be measured in a child where one or both parents have cholesterol levels ≥240 mg/dL. If their blood cholesterol is <170 mg/dL, the child is brought back in 5 years and given general risk factor and dietary advice. If the blood cholesterol level is borderline (i.e., between 170-199 mg/dL), the cholesterol is repeated and if the average cholesterol is <170 mg/dL, the child is seen again in 5 years. However, if the average cholesterol is >170 mg/dL, the child needs a lipoprotein analysis. A lipoprotein profile is indicated in all children with a high cholesterol (≥200 mg/dL).

The evaluation and follow-up recommended by the NCEP Pediatric Panel is based on the result of the average LDL cholesterol level derived from two lipoprotein profiles obtained in the fasting state at least 3 weeks apart. If the average LDL cholesterol is < 110 mg/dL, the child receives general risk factor and dietary education and returns in 5 years for repeat lipoprotein analysis. If the average LDL cholesterol level is between 110 and 129 mg/dL, the child needs more formal dietary instruction, risk factor modification, and is brought back in 1 year for a follow-up blood test. Those with an LDL cholesterol >130 mg/dL return for more detailed clinical and family assessment.

With regard to LDL cholesterol, it is clear today that it is an independent risk factor for coronary artery disease. In addition, numerous studies are now showing that lowering LDL cholesterol, either by diet alone or in combination with drug therapy, can have a beneficial effect with regard to cardiovascular morbidity and mortality and total mortality.

2.) Low Levels Of HDL Cholesterol

While a low level of HDL cholesterol is an independent risk factor for coronary artery disease in the American population, as shown clearly in the Framingham study, not all patients who have low levels of HDL cholesterol are at risk for premature atherosclerosis. For example, patients with very low levels of HDL cholesterol due to a mutation in apoprotein A-I, such as A-I Milano, do not have an increased risk for coronary artery disease. However, mild-to-moderate reductions in HDL cholesterol can result in premature atherosclerosis. Some of the more common causes of low HDL cholesterol levels include smoking, diabetes, renal disease, obesity, and certain drugs such as beta-blockers. Also, there is a familial syndrome of hypoalphalipoproteinemia where the index patient and family members have low levels of HDL cholesterol and a propensity to premature atherosclerosis.

3.) Hypertriglyceridemia

A classification of hypertriglyceridemia in adults, according to the new ATP II guidelines is as follows: normal <200 mg/dL; borderline high 200-400 mg/dL; high 400-1000 mg/dL; and very high >1000 mg/dL. While an elevated serum triglyceride is positively correlated with an increased risk for coronary artery disease in univariate analysis, this ceases to exist in multivariate analysis. The relationship between triglycerides and coronary artery disease appears to be complex and may be explained by its association with low levels of HDL and abnormal forms of LDL (e.g., small dense LDL) and elevated remnant lipoprotein levels,and a thrombogenic diathesis. However, the major problem with hypertriglyceridemia is when values exceed 1000 mg/dL (the chylomicronemia syndrome) since there is an increased risk for pancreatitis. Some of the secondary causes of hypertriglyceridemia, such as obesity, diabetes, alcoholism, renal failure, etc. are listed in Table 4. However, there are also familial forms of hypertriglyceridemia. For example, the Type IV hyperlipoproteinemia (primary endogenous hypertriglyceridemia), which is inherited as an autosomal dominant trait, results in mildly elevated triglyceride levels. This disorder manifests mainly in adulthood and does not appear to have any unique biochemical features. There is no direct evidence that these patients are more prone to coronary artery disease. These patients generally are obese and can have abnormal glucose intolerance and/or hypertension. Triglyceride levels in these patients are generally between 250 and 600 mg/dL. LDL cholesterol levels are usually normal. However, there are numerous causes of a very severe hypertriglyceridemia resulting in the chylomicronemia syndrome. In children and young adults, the chylomicronemia syndrome can be due to lipoprotein lipase deficiency which is an autosomal recessive disorder or due to a deficiency of the cofactor for lipoprotein lipase, apoprotein C-II. LPL deficiency presents in childhood with pancreatitis, eruptive xanthoma, hepatosplenomegaly and lipemia retinalis. These patients are not prone to premature atherosclerosis. Apoprotein C-II deficiency is a rare autosomal recessive disorder caused by an absence of or a defect in apo C-II, the essential co-factor for lipoprotein lipase. This results in a functional deficiency of lipoprotein lipase and an accumulation of VLDL and chylomicrons. However, the most common cause of the chylomicronemia syndrome is when it presents in adults as a Type V disorder. Generally these patients have familial hypertriglyceridemia (Type IV) and some secondary factor that triggers the chylomicronemia syndrome, such as obesity, diabetes, alcoholism etc. The type V disorder is characterized by fasting chylomicronemia and elevated VLDL levels. While the familial nature is well-recognized, the patterns of inheritance is not clear, and no specific molecular defect has been identified to date. Like patients with the Type I syndrome, with lipoprotein lipase deficiency, the Type V disorder can present with eruptive xanthoma, hepatosplenomegaly, lipemia retinalis and predisposes to pancreatitis.

The mechanism of pancreatitis with hypertriglyceridemia remains to be elucidated. It is possible that the hydrolysis of triglycerides and phospholipids results in excess lysolecithin and free fatty acids in the pancreatic bed, which function as noxious agents on the pancreatic acinar cells resulting in acute pancreatitis.

4.) Combined Hyperlipidemia

The most common familial syndrome resulting in combined hyperlipidemia is familial combined hyperlipidemia (FCHL), which is also referred to as familial multiple lipoprotein-type hyperlipidemia. In this disorder, patients and their affected first-degree relatives may at various times manifest hypercholesterolemia, hypertriglyceridemia or combined abnormalities. It also appears to be inherited in an autosomal dominant mode. To date, the underlying molecular defect has not been elucidated. However, there appears to be hepatic overproduction of apo-B containing lipoproteins that results in increased apo-B levels in VLDL, IDL and LDL. Patients usually present with hyperlipidemia in the third or fourth decade and have an increased propensity for premature atherosclerosis. This disorder may be accompanied by obesity, and abnormal glucose tolerance. The individuals may present with hypercholesterolemia, hypertriglyceridemia or combined hyperlipidemia. HDL levels are usually low in these patients. The diagnosis depends on the demonstration of multiple lipoprotein phenotypes in first-degree relatives of the patient. Apoprotein B levels are invariably elevated in these subjects. In addition, a subset of patients with premature CAD have normal LDL-cholesterol levels but elevated apo B levels, this disorder being termed hyperapobetalipoproteinemia and appears to be a subset of FCHL.

Familial dysbetalipoproteinemia or Type III hyperlipoproteinemia, which is also referred to as remnant removal disease or broad beta disease, is a rare disorder that can result in a combined hyperlipidemia. These patients usually have an abnormality in apoprotein E. Apoprotein E has 3 major alleles, apo E_{3}, apo E_2 and apo E_4. The majority of the population are homozygous for apoprotein E_3. Patients who usually get the Type III disorder are homozygous for apoprotein E_2 or have a deficiency of apo E. However, this is not sufficient to result in the Type III hyperlipoproteinemia because the frequency of E_2 homozygosity in the population is 1:100, whereas the frequency of type III dyslipidemia is 1:5,000 to 1:10,000. In addition, a secondary factor that results in overproduction of lipoproteins, such as obesity, diabetes or hypothyroidism, or a concomitant familial disorder is needed for the disorder to manifest. These patients usually present with a combined hyperlipidemia, with similar elevations in both cholesterol and triglycerides. Electrophoresis of their serum reveals a broad beta band in about 50% of patients. This is one of the rare disorders in which the basic lipoprotein profile is not sufficient and further testing, such as ultracentrifugation to quantitate the VLDL cholesterol is required. To confirm the diagnosis, the ratio of VLDL cholesterol to total plasma triglycerides should be ≥0.30 and the VLDL should exhibit beta mobility. Clinically these patients present in mid-adult life with two forms of xanthoma; 1.)xanthomas in the creases of their palms and fingers, where it imparts a yellowish discoloration, and 2.) tubero-eruptive xanthomas, which occurs at the elbows, knees and buttocks. As a consequence of accumulation of lipoprotein remnants, severe atherosclerosis of the coronary arteries and peripheral arteries can occur.

C.) Laboratory Assessment Of Dyslipidemia

In addition to a careful history and clinical examination, laboratory tests are required to establish the diagnosis of dyslipidemia and to rule out secondary causes. Either plasma or serum can be used to measure lipoprotein levels. Plasma is preferred because samples can be cooled rapidly and EDTA prevents lipid peroxidation and inhibits bacterial enzymes. Values obtained in plasma for both cholesterol and triglycerides are about 3% lower than in serum. It is important that at least two lipid estimates, preferably a week apart, be done before an individual is diagnosed as having a dyslipidemia since plasma lipids show biological variation from day to day. Reported biologic variability for total cholesterol, triglycerides, LDL cholesterol and HDL cholesterol are 6.1%, 22.6%, 9.5%, and

7.4%, respectively. According to the new guidelines of the ATP, the initial classification of hyperlipidemia in adults begins with the measurement of total and HDL cholesterol levels. The prime purpose of the HDL cholesterol measurement is to determine risk status. Both these measurements, i.e., total cholesterol and HDL cholesterol, can be obtained in the non-fasting state. Since serum is most frequently used for these measurements, serum cholesterol levels are reported in the ATP II's document. In subjects with a total cholesterol below 200 mg/dL with a concomitant HDL below 35 mg/dL, a borderline cholesterol between 200 and 239 with an HDL cholesterol below 35 mg/dL or two or more risk factors, and a total cholesterol over 240 mg/dL, a lipoprotein profile is required to determine the LDL cholesterol. The precautions that need to be undertaken prior to blood sampling include the following: 10 to 12 hour fast, avoiding alcohol on the evening prior to sampling, having been on habitual weight-maintaining diet for at least 2 to 3 weeks, lipid analysis should be deferred for 2 to 3 weeks after minor illness and for 3 months after a major illness, surgery or trauma, posture should be standardized and it is most convenient to take the sample after the patient has been seated for 5 to 10 minutes and finally drugs that affect lipid metabolism should be discontinued for at least 3 weeks, if possible. From the measurement of the total cholesterol, triglycerides and the HDL cholesterol, the LDL cholesterol can be computed. The HDL cholesterol is determined after precipitation of apo-B containing lipoproteins by polyanions and divalent cations. Using the Friedewald equation, the LDL cholesterol is computed as follows: LDL Cholesterol = Total Cholesterol - HDL Cholesterol - Triglyceride/5. This formula is not reliable if the triglycerides are over 400 mg/dL or if the rare type III hyperlipoproteinemia is suspected. Although lipoprotein electrophoresis is not recommended in the primary investigation of hyperlipidemia, it has two useful applications. It can be used to identify the broad beta band in patients with type III hyperlipoproteinemia who present with a combined hyperlipidemia to differentiate this from the more common type II-B variety which displays discrete beta and pre-beta bands. Also lipoprotein electrophoresis may prove useful to confirm the presence of chylomicrons, which remain at the origin on electrophoresis of the plasma. In subjects who have high fasting triglycerides, >500 mg/dL, the refrigerator test may prove useful in determining if VLDL, chylomicrons, or both are increased. A plasma sample is stored in a glass tube at 4 °C for 18 hours. The interpretation is as follows: if there is a turbid infranate with a creamy layer on the top, this indicates an increase in both VLDL, plus chylomicrons; if there is a clear infranate with a creamy layer on the top, this suggests increase in chylomicrons only; and finally, if there is an even turbidity throughout the sample without the creamy layer, this denotes an increase in VLDL only.

Whereas an increased level of apoprotein B, a decreased level of apoprotein A1 and a decreased apo A-1/apo B ratio have been shown to be good discriminators in identifying coronary artery disease, the addition of these assays to the present lipoprotein repertoire has not been uniformly accepted. However, much data is now accruing about the standardization of these assays and it appears that precise and accurate measurement of apoprotein B and apoprotein A-1 are available in most laboratories. As pointed out previously, the apoprotein B assay might be useful in patients with combined hyperlipidemia when the suspected diagnosis is familial combined hyperlipidemia and also, to rule out hyperapobetalipoproteinemia in a patient with normal LDL-cholesterol and CAD. In the majority of patients, measurement of the serum cholesterol, triglycerides, HDL cholesterol and determination of the LDL cholesterol by Friedewald equation will be sufficient in the workup. Rarely, beta-quantification is required using ultra-centrifugation to confirm type III hyperlipoproteinemia in which the VLDL cholesterol/triglyceride ratio is generally ≥0.3 and the VLDL exhibits beta mobility. Also in these patients, apo-E phenotyping or genotyping can be performed to determine if these subjects are homozygous for apoprotein E_2.

To confirm the type I hyperlipoproteinemia, plasma lipoprotein lipase activity can be determined following administration of heparin or lipoprotein lipase activity could be measured in adipose tissue. While both cholesterol and triglycerides can be measured either by chemical or by enzymatic methods, the majority of laboratories today are using the rapid simple automated enzymatic analyses to measure cholesterol and triglycerides, both in plasma and in HDL. Also, more recently, a direct method for the measurement of LDL cholesterol has become available and appears to be very promising, especially with hypertriglyceridemia (≥400 mg/dL) when an LDL cholesterol is required in these subjects. This direct assay would circumvent the problem when LDL cholesterol can not be reported with the Friedewald equation. Also, new direct assays for HDL-cholesterol are now available which eliminate the need for pre-treatment by performing enzymatic analysis in a system where the reaction of cholesterol in non-HDL lipoproteins is selectively inhibited. Recently, the National Cholesterol Education Program Working Group on lipoprotein measurements published their recommendation for measurement of LDL, HDL, and triglycerides. In addition to providing an acceptable goal for both accuracy (bias) and for precision (co-efficient of variation of duplicates) the investigators have reported on the goal for total error; the goals for total error for cholesterol, triglycerides, HDL cholesterol and LDL cholesterol are ≤8.9%, ≤15%, ≤22%, and ≤12%, respectively. With regard to the apolipoprotein assays, an additional lipoprotein that appears to be related to premature atherosclerosis is lipoprotein a, Lp(a). It contains a unique apoprotein a, linked by disulfide bridge to LDL to form Lp(a). Apo(a) is highly polymorphic in size and this size variation is due to varying numbers of kringle 4 units. There is an inverse correlation between the size of the apo(a) isoproprotein and Lp(a) concentrations, the largest isoprotein associated with the lowest concentration. There is considerable homology between Lp(a) and plasminogen. Lp(a) appears to be a risk factor for both coronary atherosclerosis and cerebrovascular disease. However, a few recent prospective studies have not been able to confirm this.

Much further research is needed to understand the metabolism of Lp(a), such that rational therapies can be developed. Furthermore, standardized assays are needed before Lp(a) becomes part of the routine lipoprotein repertoire. Lp(a) levels would appear to have their major indication in young subjects with clinical atherosclerosis and a normal lipoprotein profile. Finally, laboratory investigation would also be useful in ruling out the secondary hyperlipidemias. In addition to a careful history and physical examination, certain laboratory tests are useful in excluding a secondary cause of hyperlipoproteinemia. These include urinalysis (protein and glucose), plasma urea and creatinine, TSH, glucose, plasma albumen, plasma protein electrophoresis (to identify M proteins), bilirubin,and alkaline phosphatase (cholestasis), and transaminases (prior to drug therapy).

Conclusion

Presently the majority of the lipid disorders can be managed by measurement of cholesterol, triglyceride, HDL cholesterol and LDL cholesterol using the Friedewald equation or the direct immunoseparation assay for LDL-cholesterol (Table 5). In certain instances other tests are required, such as measurement of lipoprotein lipase activity, apoprotein $E\text{-}_2$ isoforms, ultracentrifugation to determine the VLDL-chol/total triglyceride ratio and lipoprotein electrophoresis to determine the broad beta band. With the new advances in lipoprotein research, it is quite possible that additional markers for premature atherosclerosis will become part of the standardized lipoprotein repertoire. For instance, the determination of Lp(a) levels, the determination of the LDL particle size by gradient gel electrophoresis, the measurement of HDL subclasses, plasma fibrinogen and homocysteine and the possible measurement of oxidizability of lipoproteins and the antioxidant status of the plasma in subjects.

Table 5. Laboratory Assesment of Dyslipidemia and CAD

A.) ROUTING TESTS:
Serum cholesterol
Serum triglycerides
Serum HDL-cholesterol
* Serum LDL-cholesterol (measured or calculated)
Tests to rule out secondary causes
B.) ADDITIONAL TESTS:
Beta quantification
Lp (a)
Apolipoprotein B
Lipoprotein Lipase Assay/Apo C-11
Apo E-genotyping
Homocysteine

**obtain LDL-cholesterol if Total cholesterol ≥ 240 mg/dl, if total cholesterol between 200-239 mg/dl with 2 CAD risk factors or HDL-C < 35 mg/dl of if total cholesterol < 200 mg/dl with HDL-C < 35 mg/dl.*

References

1. Expert Panel. Summary of the Second Report of the National Cholesterol Education Program (NCEP) Expert Panel on Detection, Evaluation, and Treatment of High Blood Cholesterol in Adults (Adult Treatment of High Blood Cholesterol in Adults (Adult Treatment panel II). JAMA 1993;269:3015-3023.
2. Jialal I. A practical approach to the laboratory diagnosis of dyslipidemia. Am J Clin Path 1996;106:128-138.
3. Thompson R. Primary hyperlipidaemia. Br Med Bul 1990;46:986-1004.
4. Jialal I. Diagnostic Tests in Endocrinology and Diabetes. Dyslipidaemias and Their Investigation. Chapman & Hall Medical, London, 1994;215-217.
5. Reed R. [Editorial]. In search of the ideal measurement of high-density lipoprotein. Clin Chem 1997;43(10):1809-1810.
6. Patsch W, Patsch JR, Gotto AM. The hyperlipoproteinemias. Med Clin North Am 1989;73:859-893.
7. National Cholesterol Education Program Report of the Expert Panel on Blood Cholesterol Levels in Children and Adolescents. Pediatrics 1992;89:(Suppl):525-584.
8. Smith SJ, Cooper GR, Myers GL, Sampson EJ. Biological variability in concentrations of serum lipids: Sources of variation among results from published studies and composite predicted values. Clin Chem 1993;39:1012-1022.
9. Bhatnager E, Durrington PN. Does measurement of apolipoproteins add to the clinical diagnosis and management of dyslipidemias? Curr Opin Lipidol 1993;4:299-304.
10. Cooper GR, Omar Henderson L, Smith JS, Hannon WH. Clinical applications and standardization of apoprotein measurements in the diagnostic workup of lipid disorders. Clin Chem 1991;37:619-620.
11. Marcovina SM, Albers JJ, Henderson LO, Hannon WH. International Federation of Clinical Chemistry Study on the Standardization of Apolipoprotein A-1 and Apolipoprotein B. Curr Opin Lipidol 1991;2:355-361.
12. Rader DJ, Brewer B. Lipoprotein(a): Clinical approach to a unique atherogenic lipoprotein. JAMA 1992;267:1109-1112.
13. Siest G, Pillot T, Bailly A, et al. Apoprotein E: An important gene

and protein to follow in laboratory medicine. Clin Chem 1995;41:1068-1086.

14. Stein EA, Meyers GL. National Cholesterol Education Program Recommendations for Triglyceride Measurement: Executive Summary. Clin Chem 1995;41:1421-1426.

15. McNamara JR, Cole TG, Contois JH, et al. Immunoseparation method for measurement of low density lipoprotein cholesterol directly from serum evaluated. Clin Chem 1995;41:232-240.

16. Jialal I, Hirany SV, Devaraj S, Sherwood TA. Comparison of immunoseparation method for direct measurement of LDL cholesterol with beta-quantification (ultracentrifugation). Am J Clin Pathol 1995;104:76-81.

17. Bachorik PS, Ross JW. National Cholesterol Education Program Recommendation for the Measurement of Low Density Lipoprotein Cholesterol: Executive Summary. Clin Chem 1995;41:1414-1420.

18. Warnick RG, Wood PD. National Cholesterol Education Program Recommendations for Measurement of High Density Lipoprotein Cholesterol: Executive Summary. Clin Chem 1995;41:1427-1433.

8

Endocrine Disorders of the Gastrointestinal Tract

RATTAN JUNEJA, MBBS., MD, MRCP &
DANIEL D. BANKSON, SM, PHD., DABCC

Gastrointestinal Disorders

Introduction

Even though the birth of endocrinology goes back one hundred years to the discovery of secretin, scientists' interests in gastrointestinal (GI) peptides grew from Pavlov's stimulation of pancreatic secretion through acidification of the intestine. Only in the last 20 years, however, have we developed a mature understanding of GI hormones. This delay is likely due to the fact that these peptides are widely distributed (not secreted from a distinct organ) and are present in very low concentrations. Recent advances have come with the development of molecular biology techniques, which have simplified hormone isolation, and more than 40 GI peptides have now been identified. The new and unique problem is that there are now many GI peptides with unknown functions, while certain specific GI physiological functions are still not associated with any peptide.

This review focuses on the common, well-established GI hormones. We review the biochemistry, physiology and specific clinical syndromes related to these hormones. Additionally we review general assay methods, normal reference ranges, and dynamic tests.

Terminology

The term gastroenteropancreatic neuroendocrine peptides (GEP-NEP) is most often used to describe all peptide hormones arising from the GI tract and pancreas, while the term GI neuroendocrine peptides (GI-NEP) usually refers to all the gut (including stomach) related peptides but does not include the pancreatic hormones. We will use the term "gut peptides" to describe both the GI-NEP and GEP-NEP.

The Gastroenteropancreatic Endocrine System and the Amine Precursor Uptake and Decarboxylation (APUD) Concept

The diffuse neuroendocrine system can be considered the body's largest endocrine organ. It is unique because it is not a single structure but a collection of specialized cells scattered throughout the body, being present in the gut, pituitary, hypothalamus, pineal, thyroid, parathyroid and placenta. These specialized cells have the capacity to secrete different peptides and amines. Pearse et al. were the first to suggest that although these cells are widely distributed in the body, they all have in common the capacity for Amine Precursor Uptake and Decarboxylation (APUD). These authors felt that because APUD cells commonly originated from neural crest (ectodermal) cells, APUD cells be called neuroendocrine cells. Now, we know that some peptide/amine producing cells derive from the endoderm, for example, cells of the gastroenteropancreatic endocrine system. The term APUD cells, therefore, is most appropriate for all cells with amine precursor uptake and decarboxylation ability. The term neuroendocrine cells, on the other hand, refer to all cells with features of both neuronal and endocrine cell, e.g., similar morphology and genetic programming.

Biologic Considerations of Gut Peptides

Structure

Gut peptides, with the exception of histamine and serotonin, are generally polypeptides. Because of structural homology they can be grouped into families (Table 1), with each family being derived from a single ancestral gene. Some peptides however cannot be categorized into any family and are therefore grouped together as orphan peptides. This structural homology is clinically important because the overproduction of one hormone can mimic some of the effects of another from the same family.

TABLE 1: STRUCTURALLY SIMILAR GUT PEPTIDES

GASTRIN FAMILY	TACHYKININ-BOMBESIN FAMILY
Gastrin	Substance P
Cholecystokinin	Gastrin releasing peptide
	Neuromedins
SECRETIN FAMILY	Neurokinins
Secretin	
Vasoactive intestinal peptide	ORPHAN PEPTIDES
Peptide histidine isoleucine	Somatostatin
Peptide histidine methionine	Neurotensin
Glucagon(enteroglucagon; glucagon-like peptides)	Galanin
	Pancreastatin
Gastric inhibitory polypeptide	Motilin
OPIOIDS	
Encephalin	
Beta endorphin	
Dysnorphins	
Adrenocorticotrophic hormone	
α Melanocyte stimulating hormone	
PANCREATIC POLYPEPTIDE FAMILY	
Pancreatic polypeptide	
Peptide YY	
Neuropeptide Y	

Distribution

In the GI tract, gut peptide hormones are produced in endocrine cells and neurons both of which are widely dispersed (Table 2). Most gut endocrine disorders are related to the overproduction of one peptide. However, conditions such as irritable bowel syndrome are thought to occur as a result of dysregulation of the activities of both the enteric and central nervous systems. In a situation of excess and abnormal production, any cell has the capacity to produce any or multiple hormones.

TABLE 2: GUT PEPTIDES: LOCALIZATION, ACTIONS AND FUNCTION

	DOMINANT SITE	ACTION MECHANISM*	PRINCIPAL FUNCTIONS
MOST CLINICALLY RELEVANT:			
Gastrin	Gastric antrum, duodenum	E/(N)	↑ Pepsin & acid secretion
Cholecystokinin	Duodenum, jejunum	E/N	↑ Pancreatic amylase secretion; ↑ Gallbladder contraction
Secretin	Duodenum, jejunum	E	↑ Pancreatic secretion (bicarbonate)
Somatostatin	Stomach, duodenum, pancreas	E/N/P	Inhibitory effects; ↓ Acid secretion; ↓ Pancreatic function
Vasoactive Intestinal peptide	Pancreas	N/(P)	Smooth muscle relaxation; ↑ Pancreatic secretion (bicarbonate)
RESEARCH RELEVANCE:			
Calcitonin gene related peptide	GI tract	N	Acid secretion/somatostatin release
Enkephalins	Stomach, duodenum, pancreas	N/(P)	Opiate-like actions; ↓ intestinal transport
Enteroglucagon	Pancreas, small intestine	(E)/(N)/(P)	Incretin (↑ insulin release); ↑ mucosal cell proliferation
Gastrin inhibitory polypeptide	Small bowel	E	↑ Intestinal secretion; Accentuates glucose mediated insulin release; Inhibits gastric acid secretion
Gastrin releasing peptide	Stomach, duodenum	N/(P)	↑ Release of gastrin & CCK
Motilin	Small bowel	E	↑ Intestinal motility
Neurotensin	Ileum	E/(P)	↓ GI smooth muscle contraction; ↓ Acid secretion
Neuropeptide Y	Small intestine	N	↓ Pancreatic secretion (bicarbonate & protein)
Pancreatic Polypeptide	Pancreas	E/(P)	↓ Pancreatic secretion (bicarbonate/ & protein)
Peptide YY	Small intestine, colon	E/(P)	↓ Pancreatic secretion (bicarbonate & protein); ↓ gallbladder contraction
Substance P	GI tract	N/(P)	GI Smooth muscle contractions

** E= Endocrine; (E)= presumptive Endocrine; N= Neurocrine; (N)= presumptive Neurocrine; P= Paracrine; (P)=presumptive Paracrine*

Formation, secretion and mechanism of action

Most active peptide hormones are formed through the processing of preprohormones. Usually only a few active forms are released by the endocrine cell; however, with endocrine tumors, increased amounts of intermediates may be released, some with biological activity.

Gut peptides are delivered to their sites of action in different ways. The classical 'hormonal' delivery is through the blood stream, being secreted in one site and transported to the site of action through blood. Some peptides have paracrine actions, being secreted into the interstitial fluid and producing effects on nearby cells, while others have neurocrine delivery, acting as neurotransmitters and neuromodulators. Gut peptides can also have autocrine effects, either stimulating or inhibiting the functions of the cell of origin. A single peptide may be delivered in more that one way, for example, somatostatin, which has both neurocrine and paracrine effects in the stomach (Table 2).

Once secreted, gut peptides bind to membrane-bound receptors. The synthesis, function and degradation of these receptors, which are proteins, are mediated by the peptide hormones themselves. Once bound to the receptor, peptide effects are mediated through secondary messengers such as intracellular calcium or adenylate cyclase.

Assay methods for Gut Peptides

Immunoassays

Over 90% of gut endocrine cells have now been identified compared with only 10% before 1970. This tremendous advance is due to the production of large quantities of pure peptides which followed the amino acid sequencing of the hormones. Subsequently, the development of sensitive (radio)immunoassays to these peptides and the use of monoclonal antibodies allowed a switch from cumbersome and poorly sensitive bioassays. Similarly, the cloning and identification of peptide hormone receptors has made it possible to develop radioreceptor assays. However, the problem of assay standardization remains as different antisera with different sensitivities and specificities are used. Results, therefore, must be compared with normals for each lab. Immunocytochemistry techniques have also improved with granule specific antibodies replacing non-specific granule stains to more accurately identify peptide producing cells.

Biochemistry of Individual Gut Peptides

GASTRIN FAMILY

Gastrin

Gastrin is both the best studied and the most clinically important gut peptide. It was discovered in 1905, but was first sequenced and synthesized only in the 1960's. It exists in three molecular forms, G-14 or mini gastrin which has 14 amino acids, G-17 or little gastrin (17 amino acids) and G-34 or big gastrin (34 amino acids). The biologically active part of the gastrin molecule is the last four amino acids of the carboxyl terminal residue which is identical in all three gastrin molecules, while the amino terminal is variable.

Secretion

Gastrin is almost entirely synthesized by the mucosa of the gastric antrum and the upper small intestine. The larger G-34 form (secreted from the intestinal G cells) has the longest half life (40 minutes) while the G-17 form (produced by the antral mucosa) has a short half life of only 5 minutes but is the predominant form in humans. Stimuli that release gastrin include:

- Presence of amino acids and breakdown products of proteins in the stomach
- Local stomach distention
- Central vagal stimulation
- To a lesser degree, calcium, alcohol and coffee

An inactive gastrin is initially released but is converted to its active form by a deaminizing enzyme. Feedback mechanisms that inhibit gastrin release include low gastric luminal pH and somatostatin (acting as a paracrine control). In atrophic gastritis, gastrin levels are very high due to lack of acid in the stomach, and a similar situation occurs following vagotomy since directly stimulated acid secretion is greatly reduced, even though vagal stimulus for gastrin release is lost.

Actions

After its release, gastrin binds to the cholecystokinin B receptor (CCKBR) which is different from the CCK A receptor (CCKAR) that binds cholecystokinin and:

- Directly stimulates the release of stomach acid
- Causes acid secretion indirectly by releasing histamine from enterochromaffin-like (ECL) cells in the gastric mucosa (H_2 antagonists completely inhibit gastrin stimulated acid secretion in vivo)
- Stimulates the release of intrinsic factor
- Stimulates mucosal blood flow
- Stimulates pepsin release
- Acts on smooth muscles and slows gastric emptying

Blood Levels

Gastrin is measured by radioimmunoassay. Being extremely labile, speci mens should be frozen promptly after centrifugation in the cold. High triglycerides may cause false increases while heparin may alter binding to resins in some assays. Different molecular weight forms show different reactivity with each antiserum, which can cause difficulties with interpretation. Physiologically, postprandially and the presence of Helicobacter pylori increase gastrin levels. Caffeine, calcium, catecholamines, insulin, omeprazole and ranitidine increase gastrin levels while atropine, lithium and octreotide reduce its levels. Fasting levels average between 21-105 pg/mL (10-50 pmol/L). These "normal" levels can be up to double the stated reference intervals in some labs. Postprandial levels (30-60 minutes after a meal) average an increase of 42-84 pg/mL (20-40 pmol/L). Besides gastrinoma (see tumor syndromes related to GI hormones), other conditions associated with raised serum gastrin levels are shown in Figure 1.

SECRETIN FAMILY

Vasoactive intestinal polypeptide (VIP)

VIP is a 28 amino acid peptide which is co-synthesized with other members of the secretin family, peptide histidine methionine (PHM) (which is secreted in humans) or peptide histidine isoleucine (PHI) (which is the non-human counterpart of PHM and is produced by other species).

Secretion

VIP occurs widely in the central and peripheral nervous systems. Significant amounts of VIP are also present in the male and female urogenital tract. Neurogenic stimuli such as stimulation of the vagus nerve or specific organs are responsible for VIP release. Once released it has a very short half-life of about 3 minutes.

FIGURE 1. GASTRIN AND STOMACH ACID OUTPUT IN THE DIAGNOSIS OF GASTRINOMA (ZOLLINGER-ELLISON SYNDROME)

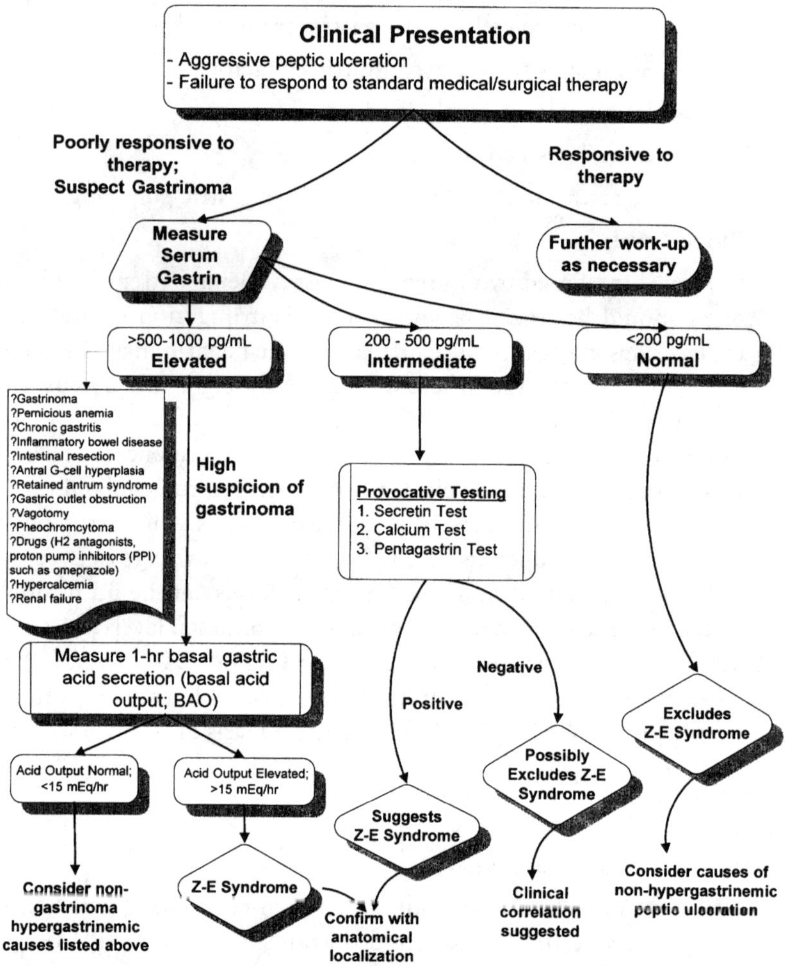

Actions

There are a large number of actions of VIP in the gut, cardiovascular, respiratory, central nervous, endocrine and immune systems. These actions are mediated by G protein activated adenylate cyclase and which of these actions is the predominant one depends on amount, rate and site of VIP administration or release.

The general actions of VIP include:

- Relaxation of vascular and nonvascular smooth muscle

- Stimulation of water, electrolyte and sometimes enzyme secretion
- Acting as a neurotransmitter/neuromodulator
- Promoting blood flow by producing vasodilation
- Stimulation of prolactin and other hypothalamic-pituitary hormone secretion
- Stimulating penile erection

In the gastrointestinal tract, VIP produces:

- Relaxation of the lower esophageal sphincter, the gastric fundus and the anal sphincter
- Inhibition of gallbladder contractility
- Increase in gut blood flow

Hypersecretion of VIP as in VIPomas (discussed later) is responsible for the chronic watery diarrhea syndrome. Hyposecretion of VIP by nerves is thought to be related to the pathogenesis of Hirschsprung's disease, achalasia of the esophagus and the high sweat Cl^- ion concentration in cystic fibrosis.

In pharmacological doses and when infused IV, VIP inhibits pentagastrin and histamine-induced gastric acid and pepsin secretion. VIP also stimulates lipolysis and glycogenolysis. Since VIP is a bronchodilator, reduced VIP (hence reduced bronchodilation) may be related to the pathogenesis of bronchial asthma.

Blood Levels

Immunofluorescence and radioimmunoassays are the primary assays used to detect VIP. Since VIP is extremely labile, samples must be collected in a pre-chilled plastic syringe containing 1.2 mg EDTA and plasma frozen immediately upon separation. Fasting serum levels are <75 pg/mL (this level is dependent on the testing laboratory due to the variability in assays). Exercise, fat ingestion, chronic renal failure and obesity all increase VIP levels, but there is no postprandial change.

Glucagon-Like Peptides and Enteroglucagon (**synonym: Glicentin; Gastrointestinal glucagon-like immunoreactivity (GLI)**)

Different forms of glucagon are found in the intestinal mucosa, stomach, salivary glands, brain and pancreas. All the glucagon molecules are derived from the same prepropolypeptide (Figure 2). The best known form is the 29 amino-acid glucagon produced by the pancreatic A cells, which has a role in glucose homeostasis. Intestinal mucosal cells produce enteroglucagon, which has the complete amino-acid sequence of pancreatic glucagon within it. The carboxy terminal flanking sequence beyond the glucagon molecule contains sequences of two more glucagon-like peptides, GLP-1 and GLP-2. Pancreatic GLP-1 inhibits gastric acid secretion and stimulates insulin secretion and like gastric inhibitory peptide (GIP), may act as an "incretin," helping to lower blood sugar in patients with type 2 diabetes. Both pancreatic GLP-1 and GLP-2 may have a role in the process of digestion other than in carbohydrate metabolism but no pharmacological actions have as yet been shown for either molecule. Enteroglucagon also inhibits gastric acid secretion but its main role is to promote mucosal growth in the intestine. The functions of the GLP's produced by the intestinal mucosal cells are unknown.

FIGURE 2: DIAGRAM OF THE ACTIVE PEPTIDES FOUND IN HUMAN PREPROGLUCAGON (AFTER BELL GI, ET AL, NATURE 1983,302:716.).

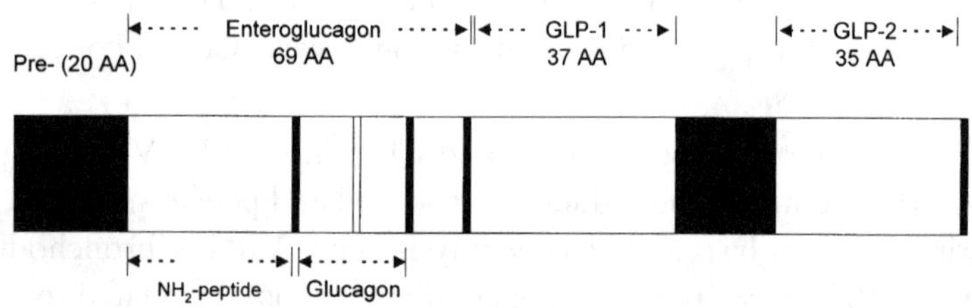

Blood Levels

Glucagon (which includes enteroglucagon) is usually measured by radioimmunoassay with fasting levels ranging from 20-200 ng/L (20-200 pg/mL). Blood should be drawn into a chilled EDTA tube, transported to the laboratory immediately and spun in a refrigerated centrifuge. Glucagon levels increase slowly following a meal, but fasting, obesity, stress, exercise and renal failure are also associated with increased levels. Immediately after a high carbohydrate meal, levels of glucagon drop. The assays for enteroglucagon are imprecise even though antisera reacting with the carboxy terminus of pancreatic glucagon do not react with enteroglucagon. In general, enteroglucagon levels are approximately five times greater than pancreatic glucagon.

ORPHAN PEPTIDES

Somatostatin

There are two naturally occurring forms of somatostatin with 14 and 28 amino acids (SS-14 and SS-28), and one 8 amino acid synthetic analogue (octreotide) which has the same biological effects but a longer half life. The 14 amino acid form was the first to be discovered in 1973. SS-14 is the predominant form in the brain, pancreas, upper gut and enteric neurons, whereas SS-28 is the predominant form in the intestinal mucosa but also occurs in the brain.

Secretion

Somatostatin is widely distributed in both the central nervous system and the GI tract. In the gut, it is mainly present in the gastric antrum, the D cells of the pancreatic islets and neurons of the myenteric plexus. A 116 amino acid preprosomatostatin molecule undergoes post-transalational processing at both the NH_2 and COOH terminals to produce somatostatin. There is reciprocity between somatostatin and gastrin release.

The stimuli for somatostatin release are:

- Meal ingestion (primary stimulus)
- Gastric acid
- Glucagon
- Growth hormone releasing hormone
- Neurotensin
- Corticotrophin releasing hormone
- Calcitonin gene-related peptide
- Gastrin releasing peptide

The inhibitors of somatostatin secretion include:

- Somatostatin itself
- Cholinergic stimulation
- Gastrin
- γ-aminobutyric acid
- Opiates

Among gut peptides, somatostatin is unique because it is delivered to target cells by endocrine, paracrine, autocrine and neurocrine routes. The plasma half-life of SS-14 is short at about 2-3 minutes while that of SS-28 is only slightly longer.

Actions

Somatostatin is the main inhibitory peptide of the gastrointestinal tract. It produces its effects through binding with five G protein coupled somatostatin receptors (SSTR1-5).

In the gut, somatostatin inhibits:

- The release and action of gastrin, CCK, secretin and VIP
- Secretion of gastric acid and pancreatic enzymes
- Secretion of water, bicarbonate, intestinal fluids and electrolytes
- Mesenteric blood flow (therefore lowers portal pressure)

Somatostatin has antitrophic (antiproliferative) effects in

- Pancreatic acinar cells
- Some neoplastic cells

Other actions of somatostatin:

Hypothalamic-pituitary axis:

- Inhibits thyrotropin releasing hormone (TRH), corticotropin releasing hormone (CRH), norepinephrine release
- Inhibits growth hormone (GH) and thyroid stimulating hormone (TSH/thyrotropin) release
- Suppresses elevated ACTH levels in Addison's disease and any ACTH producing tumor
- Reduces elevated prolactin levels in acromegaly

Thyroid:

- Inhibits T4, T3 and calcitonin release

Kidneys:

- Inhibits renin release
- Reduces anti-diuretic hormone (ADH) mediated water reabsorption

Adrenals:

- Inhibits aldosterone and catecholamine release

Blood Levels

Because of the presence of many molecular forms, rapid enzymatic degradation and widely differing radioimmunoassays, the measurement of plasma somatostatin levels is difficult. There is a 20% diurnal variation with somatostatin values increasing during the evening to peak at midnight gradually decreasing to low levels at 8:00 am. Somatostatin levels increase after meals, with renal failure, hemoconcentration and pregnancy while oral contraceptives result in decreased levels. The presence of theophyllines interfere with binding resulting in falsely low results in some assays and falsely high results in others. Plasma somatostatin (consisting of both SS-14 and SS-28) is usually reported as somatostatin like immunoreactivity (SSLI) which is <2.35 ng/dL (<10 pmol/L) in the fasting state and more than doubles postprandially.

Tumor Syndromes Related to Gut Peptides

One of the salient features of the pathology of GEP-NE tumors is that they are either associated with hyperfunction or no function but never with hormone deficiencies. Among the GEP-NE tumors, the commonest are tumors arising in the pancreas followed by intestinal tumors with gastric tumors being the least common. Within the pancreas, the most frequent functional tumor is insulinoma (discussed elsewhere in the book), while gastrinomas are the commonest malignant GEP-NE tumors. Most of these tumors are slow growing with hormone production rather than tumor bulk being responsible for the clinical manifestations. The majority of these tumors produce only one peptide hormone, but with cytotoxic treatment, can produce another peptide. Tumor cells producing inappropriate hormones are more aggressive and malignant than tumor cells producing 'eutopic' hormones, for example, pancreatic tumors composed of cells normally found in the pancreas are less malignant (e.g., insulinoma) than those producing ectopic gut hormones (e.g., gastrin, VIP). The most malignant are those that produce hormones not normally found in the pancreas or the gut (e.g., ACTH, PTH). Since many of these tumors can arise as part of the Multiple Endocrine Neoplasia (MEN) syndromes, especially MEN 1, it is important to rule out MEN in every patient with a GEP-NE tumor, since this has significant implications for both the patient and other family members. Pancreatic islet, pituitary, and parathyroid tumors characterize MEN 1.

Specific Gut Endocrine Tumor Syndromes

Gastrinoma (*synonym*: Zollinger Ellison Syndrome; Z-E Syndrome)

Epidemiology

These tumors were first described in 1955 by Zollinger and Ellison and consist of a triad of

- Islet cell tumor

- Peptic ulceration
- Failure of ulceration to respond to standard medical and surgical therapy

Gastrinomas are very rare tumors with an annual incidence of 1 per million.

Pathophysiology

Gastrinomas can be very small, 2-3 mm in size, and most commonly arise in the pancreas. About 40% of them arise in the duodenum where they are often multiple and also more malignant. When associated with MEN 1, gastrinomas again tend to be multiple. More than 50% are malignant with liver and lymph node metastasis.

Clinical Features

The Zollinger Ellison Syndrome is characterized by:

- Aggressive peptic ulceration (95% of patients); recurrent ulceration with perforation and hemorrhage, ulceration in atypical sites such as distal duodenum and jejunum, multiple ulcers.
- Hypergastrinemia
- Gastric acid hypersecretion

Five percent of patients may have diarrhea as their presenting symptom, which may precede peptic ulceration by many months. This diarrhea is mediated by acid neutralization of pancreatic enzymes, leading to a secretory diarrhea from the irritated small intestine. The peptic ulceration characteristically is either poorly responsive to standard H_2 blockade or invariably recurs despite medical therapy.

Diagnosis

An increasing awareness has resulted in earlier diagnosis of gastrinomas. However, since they are very rare, it is not economical to routinely screen for these tumors. The *sine qua non* is the finding of high serum gastrin levels in the face of high gastric acid secretion (Figure 1). It is important to emphasize that normal values for gastrin vary considerably between labs and one must always correlate results with the reference ranges set by each laboratory. If a patient with a known pancreatic tumor has recurrent aggressive peptic ulceration and a very high serum gastrin level, then the diagnosis of gastrinoma is certain and these patients will not need acid secretory studies. However, if the gastrin levels are intermediately elevated (Figure 1), then provocative tests may be needed. These provocative tests include:

A] The secretin test: This is the test of choice because it is safe, reliable, and it is easy to perform. After drawing a baseline gastrin sample, secretin is administered at a dose of 2 units/kg intravenously. Serum samples for gastrin are collected at 5-minute intervals for the next 30 minutes. Secretin normally suppresses gastrin, but in patients with gastrinoma there is a greater than 50% rise above baseline within 30 minutes of injection. An absolute rise in serum gastrin of greater than or equal to 200 pg/mL over basal levels is considered diagnostic for Zollinger Ellison syndrome. In normal individuals the increase will not be greater than a 50% rise above baseline or an absolute increase of 50 pg/mL.

B] The calcium test: Calcium gluconate is infused intravenously at the rate of 5 mg/kg/h for 3 hours. Serum samples for gastrin are collected at 30-minute intervals for 4 hours. In patients with gastrinoma, serum gastrin increases by more than 400 pg/ml above basal levels following the calcium injection.

C] The pentagastrin test: Requires measurement of basal acid output (BAO) and post pentagastrin maximal acid output (MAO). The BAO/MAO ratio is greater than 0.6 in patients with gastrinomas, since the parietal cells are near maximal stimulation in these patients and pentagastrin has little or no effect. Using a cutoff for BAO of >15 mEq/hr includes 66-99% of all Zollinger Ellison patients and excludes 90% of patients with idiopathic duodenal ulcer.

If initial testing suggests gastrinoma, anatomical localization should be attempted by CT scanning (which should include the liver to rule out metastasis), selective angiography and transhepatic portal venous sampling and sometimes surgical exploration with intraoperative ultrasonography. These localization techniques can identify up to 90% of gastrinomas.

SOMATOSTATINOMA

Epidemiology

Somatostatinomas are rare tumors with a reported incidence of 1 in 40 million. They can occasionally occur in association with neurofibromatosis (von Recklinghausen disease).

Pathophysiology

About 60% of these tumors present as a large pancreatic mass arising from the D cells, while the remaining are duodenal, usually periampullary in location.

Clinical Features

Since these tumors can become quite large in size, the majority of patients present with symptoms and signs of mass effect. Some patients may present with a clinical syndrome consisting of a triad of:

- Diabetes mellitus
- Steatorrhea
- Gallstones

The diabetes is usually mild having been present for 10 or more years. In addition, achlorhydria is a feature of somatostatinoma. All these symptoms are related to the inhibitory effects of somatostatin on insulin production, pancreatic enzyme and bicarbonate secretion, acid production, and gallbladder contractility. Some patients may have considerable weight loss, the pathophysiology of which is not known.

Diagnosis

When suspected clinically, fasting plasma somatostatin (consisting of both SS-14 and SS-28) is usually measured as somatostatin like immunoreactivity (SSLI).

VIPoma (*synonym*: Verner Morrison Syndrome; pancreatic cholera)

Epidemiology

When first described in 1958 by Verner and Morrison the VIPoma syndrome was called WDHA (watery diarrhea, hypokalemia, achlorhydria) or WDHH (watery diarrhea, hypokalemia, hypochlorhydria) syndrome to differentiate it from gastrinomas which, as already discussed, also produce diarrhea but are associated with increased acid production. With the discovery of vasoactive intestinal peptide (VIP) in 1973, these tumors came to be known as VIPomas. More recently, it has been discovered that peptide histidine methionine (PHM) which is co-secreted with VIP is also produced in large amounts by these tumors and may actually be a more important than VIP as a mediator of the diarrhea.

Pathophysiology

VIPomas occur as two types:

- Pancreatic tumors: commonest type
- Extrapancreatic (30%): ganglioneuroblastomas (observed most commonly in children), bronchogenic carcinoma, pheochromocytoma all of which can produce VIP

These tumors are poorly granulated and immunocytochemistry reveals both VIP and PHM.

Clinical Features

The average duration of symptoms is about 3 years before diagnosis. The classic triad in VIPomas is:

- Profuse watery diarrhea with dehydration
- Hypokalemia
- Achlorhydria

The diarrhea is intermittent in the early stages of the disease but becomes continuous with stool volumes up to 20 L/day as the tumor grows. The term pancreatic cholera is often used to describe this syndrome. The diarrhea is without blood or mucus and unlike the diarrhea of malabsorption, persists with fasting. Hypokalemia accompanies the diarrhea with potassium losses that can exceed 300 mEq/day producing temporary neuroparalysis and even abnormal glucose tolerance due to altered insulin sensitivity. Bicarbonate ions are also lost in the diarrhea with resultant metabolic acidosis. As already discussed, VIP in large doses also inhibits gastric acid secretion which can be low or absent, hence the achlorhydria. Other accompanying features are hypercalcemia, weight loss, and sometimes mild abdominal colic and flushing.

Diagnosis

In the differential diagnosis of chronic, secretory diarrhea one must always consider VIPoma (Figure 3) and if the clinical triad as described above is present, fasting serum VIP should be measured by radioimmunoassay. Since VIP is degraded very quickly, blood should be collected in a chilled tube with the proteolytic inhibitor, aprotinin. Plasma should be immediately separated and stored at -20 °C or lower before assay. Occasionally, high plasma VIP values are found in normal individuals due to a large molecular-weight factor, which may be a form of big VIP. Chromatographic analysis of the plasma may help in these situations. Peptide histidine methionine (PHM) can also be measured and is found to be high in patients with VIPomas. If high levels of VIP and/or PHM are found, tumor localization can be attempted with CT or MRI. Unlike gastrinomas, VIPomas are usually quite large by the time of presentation and localization is relatively easy. Sometimes the tumor cannot be found and intraop erative localization may be required.

FIGURE 3: VASOACTIVE INTESTINAL POLYPEPTIDE IN THE DIAGNOSIS OF VIPOMA.

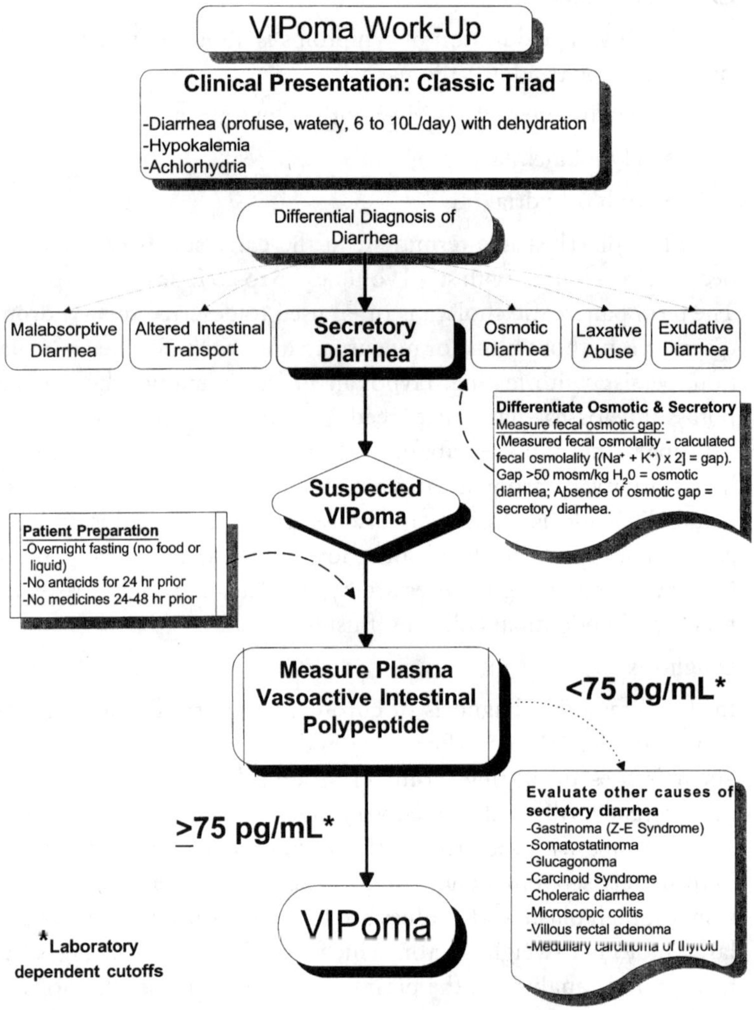

Carcinoid Syndrome (*synonym*: APUDoma's; Enterochromaffin-like (ECL) Tumor)

Epidemiology

Oberndorfer first coined the term *karzinoid* in 1907, meaning GI tumors with growth patterns like carcinomas but behaving less aggressively. In general, these tumors are rare with a reported incidence that varies with gender and age and is about 7-15 per 1 million per year. They are most common in the 5th decade. In younger patients, carcinoid syndrome is more common in women until menopause after which men are more frequently affected, suggesting the influence of hormonal factors.

Pathophysiology

ECL tumors have been reported in virtually every site in the body but most commonly arise in organs of endodermal origin, the foregut (bronchus, stomach, duodenum, jejunum, pancreas, gallbladder, ileum), midgut (appendix, colon) which is the commonest site and hindgut (rectum). Extra-gastrointestinal tumors are being detected more frequently now especially in the respiratory system. With the introduction of omeprazole, a proton pump inhibitor (PPI) for the treatment of gastroesophageal reflux disease in the 1980's, gastric carcinoids in PPI treated patients are being found with increasing frequency. The pathophysiology of PPI associated gastric carcinoids is similar to the process in pernicious anemia. These drugs produce achlorhydria, which leads to stimulation of gastrin secretion, and hence hypergastrinemia with the gastrin producing cells becoming autonomous with prolonged treatment resulting in the formation of a "hypergastrinemic" carcinoid tumor. However, these hypergastrinemic gastric carcinoids are not considered to be clinically relevant unlike gastric carcinoids in normogastrinemic patients.

Role of Serotonin (5-hydroxytryptamine, 5-HT)

Serotonin is the most common secretory product of ECL tumors. It is synthesized by enzymatic modification of circulating tryptophan by the tumors. One half of the dietary intake of tryptophan can be converted to serotonin by these cells. This leaves inadequate substrate for incorporation into proteins and niacin, precipitating protein malnutrition and pellagra.

Clinical Features

Most carcinoids remain localized and cause no symptoms due to the tumor itself. However, hormone secretion by the carcinoid cells can cause distinctive and sometimes debilitating effects, the carcinoid syndrome, which manifests with the classic triad of:

- Cutaneous flushing
- Diarrhea
- Valvular heart disease

Approximately 5% of the patients with ECL tumors experience one or more symptoms of the carcinoid syndrome. The likelihood of developing symptoms is strongly related to the site of the tumor. Thirty to sixty percent of small-bowel ECL tumors are associated with systemic manifestations, while only 3.5% of lung, 1% appendicular and virtually no rectal tumors are associated with the syndrome. In patients with intestinal tumors, humoral symptoms develop only in the setting of metastasis to the liver whereas, bronchial and other extraintestinal carcinoids where hormone products are not immediately cleared by the liver, may have the syndrome even in the absence of metastasis. Early in the course of the disease symptoms are episodic and may be provoked by stress, catecholamines, food or alcohol. Systolic blood pressure may drop 20-30 mmHg during an attack. Later, as the disease progresses the symptoms can be present most of the time.

Flushing occurs in 85% of patients with carcinoid syndrome, but only 5% of patients with new onset flushing will have the carcinoid syndrome. Other causes of flushing should be excluded before embarking on a costly work-up to rule out carcinoid. In the differential diagnosis of flushing the following conditions should be considered:

- Post-menopausal
- Drugs; Ca^{++} antagonists, Chlorpropamide plus alcohol, Antabuse treatment
- Autonomic Dysfunction; alcohol withdrawal, epilepsy
- Other Tumors; Pheochromocytoma, systemic mastocytosis (histamine release), medullary thyroid carcinoma, lymphomas, VIPoma
- Miscellaneous; Acne rosacea, mitral stenosis, anaphylaxis, idiopathic

Diarrhea may result from several mechanisms

- Mixed secretory-hypermotility induced diarrhea (most common) producing watery stools unresponsive to fasting
- Partial mechanical obstruction from tumor/fibrosis
- Mesenteric vascular insufficiency as a result of local fibrosis

Heart disease is due to endocardial fibrosis usually affecting the proximal side of the tricuspid and pulmonary valves leading to tricuspid insufficiency, pulmonic stenosis and secondary right-sided heart failure. Left-sided heart disease occurs in pulmonic tumors since the tumor products escape inactivation by lung mediators.

Diagnosis

The diagnosis of carcinoid is usually suggested by the clinical presentation (Figure 4). Measurement of 24 hour urinary 5-hydroxyindoleacetic acid (5-HIAA) is the best test. The specificity of this test approaches 100% after exclusion of substances that elevate or suppress 5-HIAA levels (Figure 4). Many patients with gastric carcinoids lack the decarboxylase enzyme that converts 5-hydroxytryptophan (5-HTP) to serotonin (5-HT). In these patients, urinary 5-HIAA can be misleading. Measuring plasma 5-HTP, histamine and urinary serotonin levels (since the kidney has the decarboxylase enzyme) helps confirm the diagnosis.

FIGURE 4: URINARY 24-HOUR 5-HYDROXYINDOLEACETIC ACID IN THE DIAGNOSIS OF CARCINOID SYNDROME.

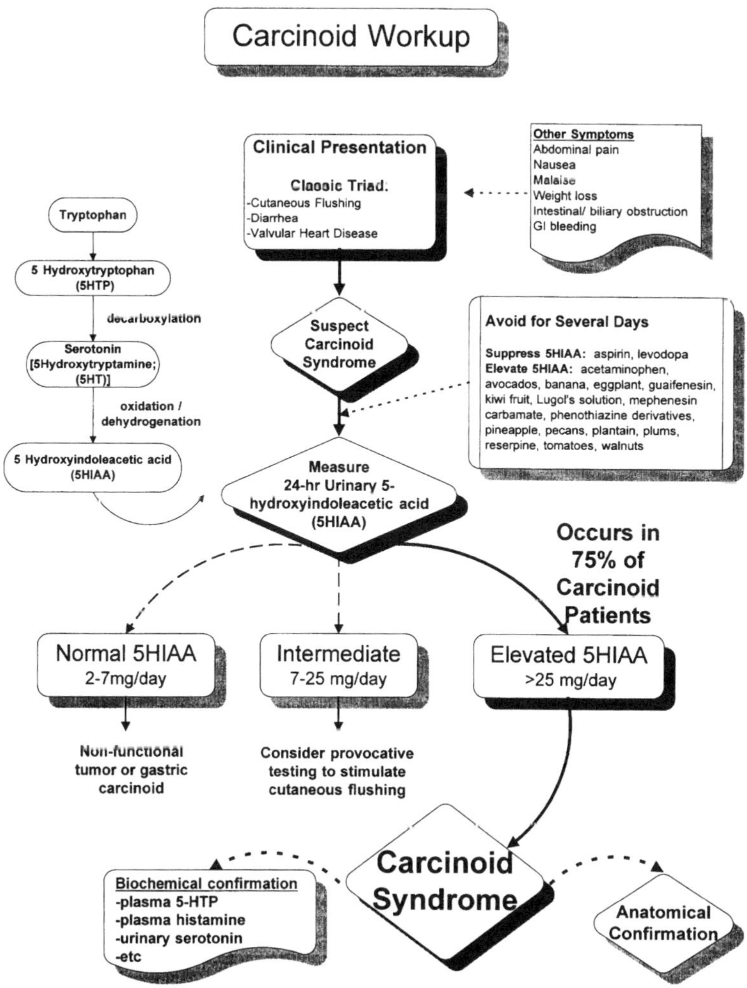

Provocative Tests: If the clinical history is equivocal, attempts to provoke cutaneous flushing may be helpful to document flushing. Ethanol, pentagastrin or epinephrine can be used for this purpose.

Anatomical Localization

Depending on the location of the tumor, endoscopy, barium studies and/or CT scan can help localize the tumor. Abdominal sonography, CT and angiography are the most sensitive ways to detect liver metastasis. Liver biopsy is the best way to obtain tissue diagnosis in patients with the carcinoid syndrome. Bone scan and echocardiography are useful detecting bone metastasis and endocardial involvement respectively. In patients where the above methods fail to localize the tumors other imaging techniques are helpful. Two more common procedures involve the use of ^{131}I-labeled Metaiodobenzylguanidine (^{131}I-MIBG) that concentrates in neuroendocrine cells and indium (^{111}In) attached to DTPA (diethylenetriaminepentaacetic acid; ^{111}In-DTPA-D-Phe; Octreotide or Pentreotide) that binds to somatostatin receptors which are expressed in large numbers by these tumors. Prognosis is inversely related to the degree of urinary 5-HIAA excretion and patients with 5-HIAA >150 mg/24 hours have a median survival of only one year. These figures were obtained prior to the advent of octreotide and interferon alpha (INF-α) treatment and survival is probably better now.

Glucagonoma

Epidemiology

Glucagonomas are rare tumors of the A cells of the pancreas with an incidence of 1 in 20 million. Eighty percent occur sporadically with a median age at diagnosis in the sixth decade. Twenty percent occur as part of the MEN 1 syndrome. Patients in the MEN-1 group tend to be diagnosed in the fourth decade.

Pathophysiology

Thirty nine percent of the tumors are found in the tail of the pancreas, 6% in the body, 11% in the head and body, while 17% are in the head alone. In 27% of cases the site of the primary tumor is never established. The majority of patients (up to 90%) have hepatic metastasis at diagnosis, especially in the right lobe of the liver.

Clinical Features

In patients with the MEN 1 syndrome, glucagonomas are usually diagnosed on routine screening before the patients become symptomatic. All patients with sporadic disease have a rash, weight loss (cachexia), diabetes mellitus (about 50% of patients) or a combination of these findings. The characteristic rash, necrolytic migratory erythema (NME), is in the form of lesions that break down with healing and residual hyperpigmentation. NME is found in over 70% of patients. Patients may also have associated glossitis and angular stomatitis. The cause of NME is unknown and it may occur in other conditions. Normochromic anemia, diarrhea, psychiatric disturbances and an increased tendency to venous thrombosis can also be present.

Diagnosis

Fasting plasma glucagon levels may be only marginally elevated (1.5 times upper limit of normal) to more than 150 times upper limit of normal in patients with glucagonoma. Thus a high index of suspicion must be maintained in patients with characteristic clinical features. In general, a fasting glucagon >200 ng/L (normal 30-200 ng/L) in the presence of characteristic clinical features is highly suggestive. Localization of the tumor can best be done with selective angiography or contrast CT scan. Preoperative localization improves clinical outcomes. Some patients with glucagonomas have an elevated fasting serum gastrin level, sometimes associated with the Zollinger-Ellison syndrome.

Conclusions

In the last decade, advances in our understanding of gut hormone physiology have produced remarkable results. The ability to measure gut peptides is useful not only to evaluate local GI/pancreatic function but also as a marker for many other conditions including certain rare tumors. Advances in receptor studies make it possible to identify naturally occurring analogues of gut peptides and to design synthetic analogues that retain the biological activity of the naturally occurring hormone and thus have tremendous therapeutic potential. The best known is the somatostatin analogue octreotide. The recognition of somatostatin receptors in various tissues and tumors has led to the development of tracer techniques, the octreotide scan, which helps to localize the tumor and to evaluate response to treatment. The potent inhibitory effects of octreotide have found therapeutic benefits in patients with metastatic gut tumors, secretory diarrhea, dumping syndrome and portal hypertension. Because of its potent bronchodilatory effects VIP may be useful in bronchial asthma (as an inhaler) and its vasodilatory effects may prove to be of benefit in male impotence and myocardial or limb ischemia. We are currently on the threshold of a new millennium, which should see increasing use of these so far elusive gut peptides both as diagnostic and as therapeutic agents. The challenge is to develop international gold standards in their measurement and to eliminate inter-laboratory variations in results.

References

1. Bayliss WM, Starling EH. Mechanism of pancreatic secretion. J. Physiol. 1902;28:325.
2. Vinik AI. A personal historical perspective of the development of the gastrointestinal endocrine system. Endocrinol. Metab. Clin. North Am. 1993;22:709-717.
3. Falkmer S. Phylogeny and ontogeny of the neuroendocrine cells of the gastrointestinal tract. Endocrinol. Metab. Clin. North Am. 1993;22:731-752.
4. Pearse AG, Takor T. Embryology of the diffuse neuroendocrine system and its relationship to the common peptides. Fed. Proc. 1979;38:2288-2294.
5. Nylen ES, Becker KL. The diffuse neuroendocrine system. In: Becker KL, ed. Principles and practice of endocrinology and metabolism. 2nd. ed. Philadelphia: J.B. Lippincott Co.; 1995:1472-1479.
6. Mulvihill SJ, Debas HT. Regulatory peptides of the gut. In: Greenspan FS, Stewler GJ, eds. Basic and Clinical Endocrinology. 5th. ed. Stamford, Connecticut: Appleton & Lange; 1997:575-594.
7. Rehfeld JF. Characteristics of diffuse peptide hormone systems. In: Becker KL, ed. Principles and practice of endocrinology and metabolism. 2nd. ed. Philadelphia: J.B. Lippincott Co.; 1995:1412-1415.
8. Holst JJ, Fahrenkrug J, Stadil F, et al. Gastrointestinal endocrinology. Scand. J. Gastroenterol. Suppl. 1996;216:27-38.
9. Bloom SR, Polak JM. The endocrine gastrointestinal tract: pathophysiology. In: Becker KL, ed. Principles and practice of endocrinology and metabolism. 2nd. ed. Philadelphia: J.B. Lippincott Company; 1995:1499-1512.
10. Walsh JH, Isenberg JI, Ansfield J, et al. Clearance and acid-stimulating action of human big and little gastrins in duodenal ulcer subjects. J. Clin. Invest. 1976;57:1125-1131.
11. Schubert ML, Makhlouf GM. Neural, hormonal, and paracrine regulation of gastrin and acid secretion. Yale J. Biol. Med. 1992;65:553-560; discussion 621-623.

12. Beinfeld MC. Cholecystokinin. In: Becker KL, ed. Principles and practice of endocrinology and metabolism. 2nd. ed. Philadelphia: J.B. Lippincott Co.; 1995:1420-1421.

13. Calam J. CCK/gastrin antagonists—clinical perspectives. Acta Gastroenterol. Belg. 1993;56:251-256.

14. Dufour DR. Reference values in endocrinology. In: Becker KL, ed. Principles and practice of endocrinology and metabolism. 2nd. ed. Philadelphia: J.B. Lippincott Co.; 1995:1957-2033.

15. Bloom SR, Hammond PJ, Polak JM. Endocrine tumors of the gastrointestinal tract. In: Becker KL, ed. Principles and practice of endocrinology and metabolism. 2 ed. Philadelphia: J.B. Lippincott Co.; 1995:1512-1518.

16. Said SI. Vasoactive intestinal peptide. In: Becker KL, ed. Principles and practice of endocrinology and metabolism. 2nd. ed. Philadelphia: J.B. Lippincott Co.; 1995:1449-1451.

17. Itoh N, Obata K, Yanaihara N, et al. Human preprovasoactive intestinal polypeptide contains a novel PHI-27-like peptide, PHM-27. Nature. 1983;304:547-549.

18. Patel YC. Somatostatin. In: Becker KL, ed. Principles and practice of endocrinology and metabolism. 2nd. ed. Philadelphia: J.B. Lippincott Co.; 1995:1436-1445.

19. Solcia E, Sessa F, Rindi G, et al. Classification and histogenesis of gastroenteropancreatic endocrine tumours. Eur. J. Clin. Invest. 1990;20 Suppl 1:S72-81.

20. White JC. Surgery of the endocrine pancreas. In: Becker KL, ed. Principles and practice of endocrinology and metabolism. 2nd. ed. Philadelphia: J.B. Lippincott Co.; 1995:1355-1360.

21. Ohneda A, Otsuki M, Fujiya H, et al. A malignant insulinoma transformed into a glucagonoma syndrome. Diabetes. 1979;28:962-969.

22. Wolfe MM, Jensen RT. Zollinger-Ellison syndrome. Current concepts in diagnosis and management. N. Engl. J. Med. 1987;317:1200-1209.

23. McGuigan JE. Peptic ulcer and gastritis. In: Isselbacher KJ, Braunwald E, Wilson JD, Martin JB, Fauchi AS, Kasper DL, eds. Harrison's Principles of Internal Medicine. 13th. ed. Vol. 2. New York: McGraw Hill, Inc.; 1994:1363-1382.

24. Verner JV, Morrison AB. Islet cell tumor and a syndrome of refractory diarrhea and hypokalemia. Am. J. Med. 1958;25:374.

25. Bloom SR, Polak JM, Pearse AG. Vasoactive intestinal peptide and watery-diarrhoea syndrome. Lancet. 1973;2:14-16.

26. Mekhjian HS, O'Dorisio TM. VIPoma syndrome. Semin. Oncol,. 1987;14:282-291.

27. Kaplan LM. Endocrine tumors of the gastrointestinal tract and pancreas. In: Isselbacher KJ, Braunwald E, Wilson JD, Martin JB, Fauchi AS, Kasper DL, eds. Harrison's Principles of Internal Medicine. 13th. ed. Vol. 2. New York: McGraw-Hill, Inc.; 1994:1535-1542.

28. Neary PC, Redmond PH, Houghton T, et al. Carcinoid disease: review of the literature. Dis. Colon. Rectum. 1997;40:349-362.

29. Janmohamed S, Bloom SR. Carcinoid tumours. Postgrad. Med. J. 1997;73:207-214.

30. Rothmund M. Carcinoid tumors—introduction. World J. Surg. 1996;20:125.

31. Bax ND, Woods HF, Batchelor A, et al. Clinical manifestations of carcinoid disease. World J. Surg. 1996;20:142-146.

32. Frankton S, Bloom SR. Gastrointestinal endocrine tumours. Glucagonomas. Baillieres Clin. Gastroenterol. 1996;10:697-705.

33. Meko JB, Norton JA. Management of patients with Zollinger-Ellison syndrome. Annu Rev Med 1995;46:395-411.

9
Malignancy-Associated Endocrine Disorders

LORI J. SOKOLL, PHD &
DANIEL W. CHAN, PHD, DABCC

Introduction

Overall, cancers of the endocrine system are relatively rare. Of the 1,228,600 new cancer cases estimated for 1998 only 1.5% are endocrine malignancies, with the majority of cases (91%) attributed to thyroid cancer (Table 1). In contrast, endocrine-related malignancies in which exogenous hormones constitute risk factors for disease or in which malignancies are responsive to hormonal treatment comprise a much greater percent of cancer cases. For example, breast and prostate cancer lead all other cancers in estimated new cases. Therefore, this chapter on malignancy-associated endocrine disorders will examine the laboratory tests, as well as the epidemiology, risk and hereditary factors, pathology, clinical features, and additional diagnostic tests for endocrine and endocrine-related cancers.

TABLE 1. ESTIMATED NEW CANCER CASES IN 1998

SITE	TOTAL # CASES	TOTAL % ALL CASES	MALE # CASES	MALE % ALL CASES	FEMALE # CASES	FEMALE % ALL CASES
Endocrine System	18,800	1.5	5,500	0.9	13,300	2.2
Thyroid	17,200	1.4	4,700	0.7	12,500	2.1
Other Endocrine	1,600	0.1	800	0.1	800	0.1
Endocrine Related						
Breast	180,300	14.7	1,600	0.2	178,700	29.7
Ovary	25,400	2.1			25,400	4.2
Prostate	184,500	15.0	184,500	29.4		
Testis	7,600	0.6	7,600	1.2		

Adapted from reference 1

Endocrine tumors can be potentially difficult to identify and may be complex to treat. Malignancies associated with some endocrine organs, such as the thyroid, do not produce clinical endocrinopathies whereas malignancies associated with other organs, such as the pancreas, can be diagnosed by measuring increased serum concentrations of pancreatic hormones if the tumor is functional. Overall, biochemical tumor markers are of value in most of the endocrine or endocrine related malignancies with respect to diagnosis of disease, progression of disease, and monitoring the effects of therapy. In general however, tumor markers are not sensitive or specific enough for screening although prostate specific antigen (PSA) has been used for early detection in conjunction with digital rectal examination, and calcitonin has been used as a screen in relatives of affected patients with familial medullary thyroid cancer (MTC). Markers for malignancy include enzymes, hormones, oncofetal antigens, carbohydrate markers, proteins, oncogene products, genetic changes, and others. The serum and urine biochemical markers, and genetic tests associated with the endocrine malignancies described in this chapter encompass many of these categories. Dynamic or provocative tests also play a role in the diagnosis and management of some malignant endocrine disorders. Pertinent dynamic tests are described in Table 2.

MULTIPLE ENDOCRINE NEOPLASIA (MEN) SYNDROMES

The three MEN syndromes (MEN-1, MEN-2A, and MEN-2B) are familial disorders inherited in an autosomal dominant fashion which are manifested by tumors, both hyperplastic and neoplastic, arising from amine precursor uptake and decarboxylation (APUD) neuroendocrine cells. Based on the combinations of endocrine tumors involved, MEN syndromes have

TABLE 2. COMMON DYNAMIC TESTS

Test	Application	Protocol	Analyte(s) Measured (Sampling Intervals)	Interpretation
Calcium-Pentagastrin Stimulation	Medullary Thyroid Cancer	2 mg/kg elemental Ca IV (1 min), 0.5 μg/kg pentagastrin IV (5 sec), supine	Calcitonin (0, 1, 3, 5, 7, 10, 15 min)	200% increase over basal concentrations suggests MTC
Clonidine Suppression	Pheochromocytoma	0.3 mg oral after overnight fast, supine	Total Catecholamines (0, 30, 60, 90, 120, 150, 180 min)	No suppression to < 500 pg/mL at 2-3 h with pheochromocytoma
Dexamethasone Suppression (Overnight - 1 mg)	Cushing syndrome	1 mg oral at 11 PM	Cortisol (8 AM)	Normals <5 μg/dL, Hypercortisolism ≥ 5 μg/dL
Dexamethasone Suppression (Overnight - 8 mg)	Cushing syndrome	8 mg oral at 11 PM	Cortisol ACTH (8 AM)	No suppression=Cushing Syndrome ACTH low - adrenal source ACTH high - non-adrenal source
Dexamethasone Suppression (Low dose)	Cushing syndrome	0.5 mg oral q6h x 2d (days 3 and 4)	Urine free cortisol (24 h collections x 4d), Cortisol and ACTH (8 AM , day 5)	Normal: UFC decreased by 50% on dexamethasone, cortisol <5 μg/dL and ACTH < 20 pg/mL; UFC ≥ 20 ug/d diagnostic of Cushing Syndrome
Dexamethasone Suppression (High dose)	Cushing syndrome	2 mg oral q6h x 2d (days 3 and 4)	Urine free cortisol (24 h collections x 4d), Cortisol and ACTH (8 AM, day 5)	Suppression UFC >50-90% of basal in Cushing disease, cortisol <5 μg/dL; no suppression: elevated ACTH=ectopic ACTH/CRH, normal/low ACTH=adrenal tumor
Glucagon Stimulation	Insulinoma	1 mg/10 mL saline IV (30 min)	Insulin (0, 1, 3, 5, 10, 20, 30 min)	Normal peak < 130 μU/mL
Secretin Stimulation	Gastrinoma	2 U/kg IV bolus	Gastrin (0, 2, 5, 10, 15, 20 25, 30 min)	Increase ≥ 50% over basal in gastrinoma
Tolbutamide Tolerance	Insulinoma	1 g IV bolus	Glucose Insulin (0, 2, 15, 30, 60, 120 min)	Glucose: 50% of baseline at 30 min, return to baseline at 120 min and Insulin: peak at 2 min, <150 μIU/mL in normals

been classified as either MEN-1 or MEN-2. MEN-1 has been mapped to the long arm of chromosome 11 (11q13) and MTC that is part of MEN-2 has been mapped to the centromeric region of chromosome 10. This has allowed genetic testing of family members which, in conjunction with biochemical measurements and clinical observations, allows for screening and potential early detection of disease.

MEN-1(Wermer's Syndrome)

Epidemiology. MEN-1 is a very rare disease which occurs in 3-20 out of 100,000 individuals. Clinical manifestations usually develop in the third or fourth decade, however early diagnosis has been possible with screening.

Risk and Inheritance Factors. The gene for MEN-1, located on chromosome 11q13, was cloned in 1997. The gene encodes a 610 amino acid protein, menin, the function of which is unknown. MEN-1 has an autosomal dominant inheritance pattern. The gene appears to be a tumor suppressor gene in which tumorigenesis results from the loss of the wild-type allele in combination with the altered inherited allele (two hit hypothesis). In addition to germ-line mutations, somatic mutations have been found in sporadic tumors. Risk for MEN-1 is increased in patients with Zollinger-Ellison syndrome, insulinoma, or hyperparathyroidism. Both sexes are affected equally.

Characterization. Specific characteristics associated with MEN-1 are listed in Table 3. The parathyroid, pancreatic islet cells, and the pituitary are primarily affected, although the presentation of the disease varies among individuals, contributing to underdiagnosis of the disease. The majority of tumors are benign, with malignant tumors limited to the pancreatic islets. The parathyroid gland is involved in 90% of cases. Hyperparathyroidism, resulting from multiglandular nodular hyperplasia is often one of the first indicators of this disease. Hyperparathyroidism is commonly discovered in the second decade of life when screening family members of affected MEN-1 individuals. In adults, hyperparathyroidism is often discovered biochemically when MEN is suspected or upon additional testing when pituitary or pancreatic disease is found.

Pancreatic islet cell tumors are a manifestation of MEN-1 in 30-80% of cases. The most common tumors are gastrinomas (60%), characterized as small, multiple adenomas located in the pancreas or duodenum. A smaller percentage of gastrinomas associated with MEN-1 are malignant compared to sporadic tumors. Other pancreatic tumors found in

Table 3. Characterization of Multiple Endocrine Neoplasia

MEN-1

- Parathyroid Hyperplasia (90-97%)
- Pancreatic Islet Cell Tumors (30-80%)
  - Gastrinoma
  - Insulinoma
  - VIPoma
  - Glucagonoma
  - PPoma
  - GRFoma
- Pituitary Tumors (15-50%)
  - Prolactinoma
  - ACTH Producing Adenoma
  - Growth Hormone Secreting Tumor
  - Nonfunctioning Adenoma
- Other Tumors
  - Carcinoid Tumors
  - Adrenal Cortical Adenomas
  - Thyroid Adenomas
  - Lipomas

MEN-2

- MEN-2A
  - Medullary Thyroid Carcinoma (100%)
  - Pheochromocytoma (50%)
  - Parathyroid Hyperplasia (30%)
  - Normal Phenotype
- MEN-2B
  - Medullary Thyroid Carcinoma (100%)
  - Pheochromocytoma (50%)
  - Multiple Mucosal Ganglioneuromas (lips, tongue, eyelid)
  - Marfanoid Body Habitus

MEN-1 include: insulinomas, VIPomas (vasoactive intestinal peptidomas), glucagonomas, PPomas (pancreatic polypeptidomas), and GRFomas (growth hormone releasing factoromas). More than one type of tumor may be present in the same patient.

Pituitary tumors, another feature of MEN-1, are present in 15-50% of cases. Most pituitary adenomas are functional and commonly secrete prolactin. Growth hormone and ACTH are secreted less frequently, and elevated concentrations result in acromegaly or Cushing disease. Tumors may also be non-functional. In addition to the parathyroid, pancreatic, and pituitary involvement in MEN-1, patients have an increased frequency of adrenal cortical hyperplasia or adenomas, carcinoid tumors in the thymus (men primarily) and bronchus (women primarily), lipomas, and thyroid adenomas.

Diagnostic and Screening Laboratory Tests: Patients diagnosed with hyperparathyroidism (multiglandular disease or hyperplasia), Zollinger-Ellison syndrome, or insulinoma may be at increased risk for MEN-1 and thus should be questioned regarding a family history of MEN-1. Since the recent discovery of the MEN-1 gene, limited direct genetic testing has become available. Currently, 47 mutations of the MEN-1 gene have been identified and 85% of mutations can be detected using SSCP (single strand conformation polymorphism) analysis. Following SSCP analysis, confirmation is usually performed with a different technique. A negative test does not guarantee the lack of the disease, however. In the absence of or in conjunction with genetic testing, diagnoses can be made on the basis of clinical presentation and elevated laboratory values. History and physical exams should focus on signs and symptoms of hypercalcemia, peptic ulcer disease, hypoglycemia, galactorrhea-amenorrhea, Cushing disease, hypopituitarism, and acromegaly. Biochemical screening tests recommended to be most effective in identifying the endocrine abnormalities most common to MEN-1 include: serum calcium (albumin corrected or ionized), PTH (parathyroid hormone), prolactin, somatomedin C (IGF-1), gastrin, glucose, insulin, glucagon, and pancreatic polypeptide measurements. Measurement of these tests gives the highest yield since they screen for the most common manifestations of MEN-1. Pancreatic polypeptide concentrations can prove useful to diagnose secreting pancreatic endocrine tumors since pancreatic polypeptide tumors do not typically produce clinical symptoms. This combination of tests may be indicated when screening patients with a high suspicion of MEN-1 due to family history, multiple lesions, or positive genetic familial screening. Measurement of serum calcium, gastrin, and prolactin only may be sufficient in asymptomatic patients and patients without a positive family history. Even after initial treatment, usually surgical, regular biochemical screening, in additional to physical examination, radiological testing and other imaging studies, is required in order to detect new and recurrent tumors. Yearly biochemical screening is usually recommended.

Once a diagnosis of MEN-1 is made it is prudent to screen family members of the proband. If the mutation can be determined, family members can be screened to identify gene carriers. Prior to cloning the gene, the only available genetic testing was an indirect linkage analysis approach using polymorphic markers flanking the MEN-1 locus. This required DNA from 2 affected and 2 unaffected family members. The age at which to screen family members with genetic tests has not been agreed upon. Regular biochemical screening is advised for identified gene carriers and for family members in which genetic testing is not possible in order to detect early evidence of disease and potentially decrease morbidity and mortality. Recommended intervals of testing vary from 1 to 5 years. The most frequently detected abnormality is asymptomatic hyperparathyroidism, diagnosed from elevated serum calcium determinations.

MEN-2

Epidemiology. MEN-2A and MEN-2B are rare diseases. One thousand patients, primarily at-risk family members, are diagnosed per year.

Risk and Inheritance Factors. MEN-2A, MEN-2B, and non-MEN familial medullary thyroid cancer (FMTC) are associated with mutations of the *RET* (Rearranged during Transfection) proto-oncogene, a dominant oncogene at chromosome 10q11.2. The *RET* proto oncogene is a receptor tyrosine kinase. Receptor tyrosine kinases are found on cell surfaces and transduce signals for cell growth and differentiation. In MEN-2A and non-MEN familial MTC, point mutations are found in one of five specific cysteine residues in the *RET* extracellular domain (exons 10 and 11) while in MEN-2B there is a point mutation in the ligand-binding domain (exon 16). Ninety-five to ninety-seven percent of MEN-2A and 93-95% of MEN-2B families have been determined to have these specific mutations. *RET* mutations have also been found in sporadic disease (MTC and pheochromocytoma) and in Hirschsprung's disease, a congenital disease manifested by aganglionic megacolon. Men and women are equally affected and penetrance is age-related.

Characterization. Specific characteristics associated with MEN-2 are listed in Table 3. MEN-2A and MEN-2B are similar in some respects, yet also have distinct characteristics. In both syndromes, all patients develop MTC and approximately half develop pheochromocytomas. Thyroid C-cell and adrenal chromaffin cell hyperplasias precede the development of multifocal clonal tumors. In contrast, 20-30% of MEN-2A patients develop parathyroid adenomas and thus hyperparathyroidism. Parathyroid involvement is rare in MEN-2B. MEN-2B patients however, have a distinctive physical appearance not found in MEN-2A. Neural defects include mucosal ganglioneuromas of the lips, eyelids and tongue. An additional distinctive physical feature is a marfanoid habitus with excessive limb length, hyperflexible joints, scoliosis, and anterior chest wall deformities. Neural abnormalities may be present in the GI with the presence of ganglioneuromatosis. This may affect motility of the gut resulting in diarrhea, constipation, or a clinical picture of megacolon.

MTC differs in peak incidence between MEN-2A and MEN-2B with peaks in the second and third decades for MEN-2A and peaks in the first and second decades for MEN-2B. MEN-2B tumors are also more aggressive. In contrast to sporadic MTC tumors which are single and unilateral, familial forms are multifocal and bilateral. A thyroid nodule, goiter, mass, or cervical lymphadenopathy is present in a third of MEN-2 patients. Cushing syndrome, from ACTH secretion, and diarrhea or flushing, manifestations of excessive hormone production or tumor secretions, may be present. The majority of MTC cases are detected in asymptomatic high risk relatives through screening procedures.

Pheochromocytomas typically appear after thyroid disease in the fourth and fifth decades. Malignant tumors are rare. Although benign, severe hypertension, stroke, myocardial infarction, or death may result if untreated. In contrast to the sporadic forms of pheochromocytoma, epinephrine appears to be the dominant catecholamine produced, resulting in a lower urinary norepinephrine to epinephrine ratio. In familial disease sustained hypertension is unusual with early symptoms of anxiety, palpitations and tachycardia, and later symptoms of headache, pallor, and perspiration.

Diagnostic and Screening Laboratory Tests: Patients with MTC or pheochromocytoma should be investigated for the presence of MEN-2 syndromes since MEN is often discovered in a family following diagnosis of either of these conditions. Forty percent of MEN-2A carriers do not have symptoms thus a negative family history does not rule out the presence of the syndrome. Physical characteristics of MEN-2B allows a diagnosis on physical examination alone. MEN-2A diagnoses can be made with biochemical or genetic testing. Briefly, biochemical testing for MTC (Table 2) consists of measurement of serum calcitonin, usually following calcium-pentagastrin stimulation, since 27% of patients may have normal basal concentrations of plasma calcitonin. Testing for pheochromocytoma consists of measurement of urinary epinephrine, norepinephrine and total metanephrines, and testing for hyperparathyroidism requires measurement of serum calcium concentrations.

Prior to the discovery of the relationship between MEN-2 and the *RET* proto-oncogene, and the subsequent development of genetic tests, typical screening in MEN-2A necessitated yearly calcium-pentagastrin stimulation tests between ages 5 and 40 in addition to urinary catecholamine and serum calcium measurements. By age 40, MTC is detected in greater than 95% of cases. Using this approach, calcium-pentagastrin stimulation tests were commonly abnormal by ages 8 or 9 in gene carriers. Subsequently, total thyroidectomy resulted in over a 90% cure rate. Currently, this approach has been largely been replaced with genetic screening. There are obvious advantages to genetic testing for at-risk individuals compared to the biochemical approach including one time testing, often at birth, and elimination of the yearly and often unpleasant provocative testing. In addition, in MTC metastases may already be present at the point when the stimulation tests become positive and conversely cancer may be present in patients with a negative test result.

Mutations in the *RET* proto-oncogene in index cases and gene carriers in families at risk can be identified by direct germ-line DNA testing using a number of different techniques such as restriction enzyme cleavage based analysis, SSCP, allele specific oligoneucleotides, denaturing gradient gel electrophoresis, chemical cleavage mismatch, and heteroduplex formation. Due to the clustering of mutations, direct sequencing is also possible. Confirmation testing is not required with this technique. The majority of MEN-2A families have one of the 5 missense mutations and the majority of MEN-2B families have the single identified mutation. If a mutation in the proband is not identified, linkage analysis can predict the risk for other family members if such testing is possible. If not, continued biochemical and clinical screening is advised on an annual basis. Thyroidectomies in identified gene carries have been recommended by age 6 in MEN-2A and by age 2 in MEN-2B where MTC occurs at an earlier age and is present in a more aggressive form. These patients are then monitored for recurrence with calcium-pentagastrin stimulation testing and for development of pheochromocytomas or hyperparathyroidism starting in adolescence.

Gastrointestinal Endocrine Tumors

Gastrointestinal and carcinoid malignancies are briefly presented here and in more detail in chapters 6 and 8.

Carcinoid Tumors

A description of carcinoid tumors is found in the Gastrointestinal Endocrine Disorders chapter.

Gastrinoma (Zollinger-Ellison syndrome)

Epidemiology: Gastrinomas are rare with an incidence of 1 per million. Zollinger-Ellison Syndrome may account for 0.1% of patients with duodenal ulcer disease. Gastrinomas are the most common hormone secreting malignant pancreatic tumors.

Risk and Hereditary Factors: Thirty to fifty percent of tumors are associated with the MEN-1 syndrome.

Pathology: Sixty to seventy percent of tumors are malignant. Metastases are to the liver and lymph nodes.

Clinical Features and Laboratory Tests. Laboratory testing associated with diagnosis of gastrinoma includes serum gastrin measurements, and calcium or secretin stimulation tests (Table 2) if required. Serum gastrin concentrations >500 pg/mL are suggestive of disease and concentrations >1000 pg/mL with corresponding gastric acid hypersecretion are diagnostic. A more complete description of gastrinoma diagnosis and the clinical presentation of the disease are found in the Gastrointestinal Endocrine Disorders chapter.

Glucagonoma

Epidemiology. Glucagonomas have an incidence of 1 in 20 million per year with a peak incidence between ages 40 and 60.

Risk and Hereditary Factors. Thirty to fifty percent of glucagonomas are associated with MEN-1.

Pathology. Tumors, found in the islet A cells of the pancreas, are large and slow growing. Seventy five percent are malignant and 75% are metastatic at diagnosis. The tumors can result in elevated levels of peptides such as pancreatic polypeptide, gastrin, somatostatin, and insulin, in addition to glucagon.

Clinical Features and Laboratory Tests. Fasting plasma glucagon concentrations greater than 1000 pg/mL, in addition to characteristic clinical features (see chapter 8) are diagnostic. Hypercalcemia and hypoaminoacidemia (alanine, glycine, and serine concentrations <25% of normal) may also be present.

Insulinoma

Epidemiology: Insulinomas, the most common islet cell tumors of the endocrine pancreas, have an incidence of 4 per million per year with the largest incidence between ages 40 and 60 years.

Risk and Hereditary Factors: The majority of tumors are sporadic while 10% occur in association with MEN-1.

Pathology: Ninety-nine percent of tumors arise in the β cells of the pancreas and 80% are hormonally functional. Ten percent of tumors are malignant although slow growing. Fifty percent of patients have metastases at diagnosis, primarily to the liver and regional lymph nodes.

Clinical Features and Laboratory Tests: The diagnosis of hypoglycemia (Whipple's triad) and the diagnostic workup for the causes of hypoglycemia are described in chapter 6. The diagnosis of insulinoma is aided by measurements and observations made during a supervised prolonged fast. During the fast, patients with insulinoma will develop neuroglycopenic symptoms resulting from glucose concentrations <40 mg/dL. Concurrently, serum insulin concentrations will typically reach concentrations >6 μIU/mL and the insulin to glucose ratio will be >0.3. Similar to insulin, C-peptide concentrations will not be suppressed with hypoglycemia. Proinsulin concentrations greater than 22-25% of plasma insulin immunoreactivity are also present in insulinoma. Provocative tests demonstrating increased secretion of insulin are used on occasion in insulinoma diagnosis when other studies are borderline, and to monitor treatment response in malignant insulinomas. These provocative tests include tolbutamide tolerance and glucagon stimulation tests (table 2).

Somatostatinoma

Epidemiology. Somatostatinomas are exceedingly rare, with an incidence of 1 in 40 million. Only 60 cases have been reported in the literature.

Risk and Hereditary Factors. Tumors can be associated with von Recklinghausen's neurofibromatosis.

Pathology. Sixty percent of tumors are located in the D cells of the pancreas (50% head, 25% tail) with the majority of others located in the small intestine. Eighty percent of pancreatic and 50% of intestinal tumors are malignant. Most tumors are large and metastases are present in the majority of cases at diagnosis.

Clinical Features and Laboratory Tests. Plasma somatostatin concentrations can confirm the diagnosis of somatostatinoma. More detail on somatostatinomas can be found in chapter 8.

VIPoma (Vasoactive Intestinal Polypeptide) - Verner-Morrison Syndrome

Epidemiology. VIPoma, also referred to as pancreatic cholera syndrome or WDHA syndrome (watery diarrhea, hypokalemia, achlorhydria or hypochlorhydria), has an incidence of 1 in 10 million.

Pathology. The majority of tumors occur in the pancreatic body or tail (islet D_1 cells). Fifty percent of tumors are malignant.

Clinical Features and Laboratory Tests. In addition to characteristic clinical features, serum VIP concentrations can aid in VIPoma diagnosis. VIPoma is described in more detail in the chapter on Gastrointestinal Endocrine Disorders.

Adrenal Tumors

Adrenal Carcinoma

Epidemiology. Adrenal carcinoma is rare with an incidence of 2 per million. Incidence peaks are in children less than 5 years of age and between ages 40 and 50. Two-thirds of occurrences are in women.

Pathology. The majority of tumors are sporadic although adrenal cancer occasionally occurs in familial cancer syndromes. Fifty percent of tumors are functional, producing cortisol and other steroids. Tumors are highly aggressive. Fifty percent of patients have metastases at diagnosis, primarily to lymph nodes, lung, liver, and bone.

Clinical Features. In patients with non-functioning tumors, abdominal masses are often discovered in patients with abdominal pain and with symptoms of weight loss, fullness, indigestion, nausea, vomiting, pain, or weakness. In patients with functioning tumors, symptoms of non-functioning tumors plus those due to excess hormone and glucocorticoid secretion may be present. Features associated with Cushing syndrome are described in chapter 3. Virilization, or hirsutism in women, and feminization in men, may be present; mineralocorticoid secretion is rare. Thirty to forty percent of patients have Cushing syndrome, 20-30% have virilization, 10-30% have both, 15% have feminization, and <5% have pure hyperaldosteronism.

Laboratory Tests. A detailed description of the diagnosis of Cushing syndrome can be found in chapter 3. In summary, with an adrenal tumor, plasma ACTH concentrations are low and serum cortisol and urinary free cortisol fail to suppress adequately during the high dose dexamethasone suppression test (Table 2). Malignant, but not benign, tumors may produce steroids other than cortisol due to partial enzyme deficiencies in steroid biosynthesis pathways. Therefore, increased urinary 17-ketosteroid excretion and increased plasma DHEAS (dehyroepiandrosterone sulfate) concentrations are diagnostic of carcinoma. 17-Ketosteroids are also useful for following treatment. In women with symptoms of virilization, concentrations of plasma testosterone and androstenedione may be elevated while in men with feminization plasma estrone and estradiol may be elevated. Hyperaldosteronism will be manifested by increased plasma aldosterone concentrations.

Tumor Imaging. Adrenal tumors are often incidental findings on radiology studies or CT scans. Large tumors > 4 cm are suggestive of carcinoma.

Other Tests. Biopsies may also play a role in diagnosis.

Neuroblastoma

Epidemiology. The incidence of neuroblastoma in children is 2-10 cases per million. Sixty percent of tumors are diagnosed before age 3 and ninety percent before age 5. The incidence is rare over age 14. Neuroblastoma is the most common solid tumor malignancy in childhood.

Risk and Inheritance Factors. Neuroblastoma is more common in whites than in blacks.

Pathology. Neuroblastomas are neural crest in origin and arise from sympathetic or adrenal neuroblasts. Eighty percent of primary tumors occur in the adrenal gland or paraspinal sympathetic ganglia. Tumors grow rapidly and are highly malignant with widespread metastases to the liver, bone, skin and bone marrow.

Clinical Features. Adrenal tumors produce abdominal masses and may result in abdominal pain and distension. Other non-specific symptoms include: anorexia, fever, diarrhea, and bone pain. One in 5 patients is hypertensive; secretion of inactive catecholamine precursors as opposed to more active forms may be the explanation.

Laboratory Tests. The majority of tumors produce increased amounts of catecholamines and their metabolites which can be measured in urine and used for diagnosis as well as for monitoring treatment. Norepinephrine,

VMA (vanillylmandelic acid), HVA (homovannilic acid) may have increased excretion with increased excretion of dopamine more specific for neuroblastoma. The ratio of urinary VMA to HVA, indirectly reflecting dopamine hydroxylase, is indicative of a worse prognosis when the ratio is <1.5. Neuron-specific enolase (NSE), a glycolytic enzyme found in tumors associated with neurodendocrine origin, is elevated in greater than 90% of children with advanced disease. Levels appear to correlate with the stage of the disease and higher concentrations are indicative of a poorer prognosis. Use of NSE for monitoring is controversial.

Other Tests. Other clinical tests performed in the evaluation of neuroblastoma include bilateral bone marrow aspirates and biopsies for metastases.

Tumor Imaging. MIBG (metaiodobenzylguanidine) is a compound that resembles norepinephine and therefore can be taken up into neurosecretory storage vessels. Labeling with ^{131}I allows identification of primary and metastatic tumor sites following injection. MIBG scintigraphy is approximately 90% sensitive and 100% specific for neuroblastoma. CT or MRI scans are also employed for tumor localization.

Pheochromocytoma

Epidemiology. Pheochromocytomas are very rare except when associated with familial disease. The incidence is 0.04 per 100,000 per year. Diagnoses are most commonly made in the fourth and fifth decades and 10 percent of patients are children. Pheochromocytomas are one of most common childhood endocrine tumors.

Risk and Hereditary Factors. Pheochromocytomas are associated with hereditary syndromes in 5 to 10% of cases, such as MEN-2 and others (see chapter 3).

Pathology. Tumors are neuroectodermal in origin with 90% arising in the adrenal medulla (10% in both glands) and 10% arising in the paraganglia of the sympathetic nervous system. In addition to secreting the catecholamines epinephrine, norepinephrine, and occasionally dopamine, tumors may also secrete VIP, opioid peptides, melanocyte stimulating hormone, parathyroid-like hormone, serotonin, calcitonin, ACTH, somatostatin, and neuropeptide Y. Ten percent of tumors are malignant, but slow growing; 30-40% of extradrenal tumors are malignant. Metastases (10% of cases) are found in bone, liver, lung, and soft tissues.

Clinical Features and Laboratory Tests. See chapter 3 and table 2 for a complete description of the clinical features and diagnostic laboratory tests for pheochromocytomas. An additional laboratory test to specifically aid in the pathologically difficult diagnosis of malignant tumors is the neuroendocrine serum tumor marker NSE (neuron specific enolase). Benign tumors have not been shown to produce this marker.

Tumor Imaging: Tumor imaging is accomplished with CT scans, MRI, selective venography, and scintigraphy with ^{131}I MIBI (metaiodobenzylguanidine).

Parathyroid and Thyroid Tumors

Parathyroid

Epidemiology. Parathyroid carcinoma is very rare. Less than 0.5% of hyperparathyroidism is attributable to parathyroid malignancy. The mean age at diagnosis is 45 with equal distributions between men and women.

Risk and Hereditary Factors. Parathyroid cancer may be may be associated with familial hyperparathyroidism, MEN-1 syndromes, and external radiation.

Pathology. Less than 5% of parathyroid tumors are malignant. Tumors are slow growing with local recurrences. Metastases (uncommon) are to the bone, liver, and lung. Ninety-five percent of tumors are functional.

Clinical Features. A palpable neck lesion in the setting of hyperparathyroidism is suggestive of parathyroid cancer. Thirty to fifty percent of lesions are palpable and diagnosis is made by biopsy in combination with hyperparathyroidism. Symptoms are a result of primary hyperparathyroidism and resulting high serum calcium concentrations. Bone effects (50% of patients) include: osteitis fibrosa cystica, osteopenia, pathologic fractures, and bone pain. Renal effects (60% of patients) include: nephrolithiasis, nephrocalcinosis, polyuria, polydipsia, and decreased renal function. Neuromuscular effects include: muscle weakness and aches, easy fatiguability, paraesthesia, and mental disturbances. Rheumatologic symptoms include: joint pain, gout, and pseudogout. GI symptoms include: anorexia, nausea, vomiting, constipation, and peptic ulcers. Cardiovascular effects include calcification of the cornea and other soft tissues.

Laboratory Tests. Laboratory testing for parathyroid carcinoma reflects the presentation of hyperparathyroidism and thus focuses on serum calcium and serum PTH (parathyroid hormone) measurements. In benign causes of hyperparathyroidism serum calcium concentrations are typically in the range of 10-11 mg/dL while in malignant causes concentrations are typically higher, in the range of 15-16 mg/dL. Associated intact PTH concentrations are also markedly above the reference range (10-65 pg/mL).

Other manifestations of hyperparathyroidism include increased urine calcium excretion (>250 mg/d) and decreased urinary phosphorus excretion as well as hypomagnesemia and hypokalemia.

Tumor Imaging. Parathyroid tumors can be imaged with ultrasonography, and CT scans are employed to detect metastases.

Thyroid Cancer

Epidemiology. 17,200 new cases of thyroid cancer and 1,200 deaths from thyroid cancer are projected for 1998. Thyroid cancer is overwhelmingly the most common endocrine malignancy. Women account for 75% of cases. In familial medullary thyroid cancer (FMTC) the peak incidence is between ages 10 and 30 while the peak incidence is between ages 40 and 60 for sporadic MTC.

Risk and Hereditary Factors. The risk of thyroid cancer increases with age and can result from chronic elevations of thyroid stimulating hormone (TSH). A major risk factor is exposure to radiation, either through fallout or therapy for benign conditions. Five to 10% of irradiated individuals develop cancer, primarily papillary, and 4 to 9% of cancer patients have a history of neck radiation. Twenty percent of medullary thyroid cancer is familial, resulting from either MEN-2A, MEN-2B syndromes or FMTC. The MEN-2 syndromes and FMTC are inherited in an autosomal dominant fashion. All three result from mutations of the *RET* proto-oncogene on chromosome 10. MEN-2A and FMTC mutations (95-97%) are in one of 5 cysteine residues in exons 10 and 11.The MEN-2B mutation (93-95%) is a point mutation at codon 918 in exon 16. A point mutation has also been identified in the *ras* oncogene in 40-50% of follicular carcinomas (34).

Pathology. The most common forms of thyroid cancer are papillary carcinoma (60-70% of cases) and follicular carcinoma (15-20% of cases). Papillary tumors are the predominant form resulting from radiation exposure. Medullary carcinoma, arising from the parafollicular calcitonin secreting C cells, comprises 5-7% of thyroid malignancies. The sporadic form of the disease is typically unilateral in presentation while hereditary forms are bilateral. In familial forms, the transformation to MTC is preceded by C-cell hyperplasia. Anaplastic giant and spindle cell, and Hurtle cell carcinomas are aggressive forms of thyroid cancer accounting for 5% of cancers, while other tumors such as Hodgkin's disease, lymphomas, and soft tissue sarcomas may also be found in the thyroid.

Clinical Features. The majority of patients with thyroid cancer have no significant symptoms. Occasionally an enlarging neck mass may be present as well as hoarseness, neck pain, or dysphagia. Thyroid masses may be discovered during physical examination. Most cancerous lesions are single nodules with a hard consistency and fixation. Features specific to MTC include: secretory diarrhea in 30% of patients, seen in advanced disease, resulting from intestinal electrolyte disturbances caused by high circulating calcitonin concentrations, flushing, resulting from secretions of prostaglandins and serotonin, and Cushing syndrome as a result of tumor ACTH secretion.

Laboratory Tests. Most patients with thyroid cancer are euthyroid (normal TSH, T_4 and T_3 concentrations) and therefore thyroid function tests are not useful for diagnosing thyroid cancer. However, following treatment, ultrasensitive TSH concentrations are measured to monitor thyroid hormone therapy. Thyroglobulin concentrations are also employed following surgery or radioactive iodine ablation to detect recurrence in papillary and follicular, but not medullary thyroid cancer. Calcitonin is the most important tumor marker for the C-cell derived medullary thyroid cancers. Thyroglobulin is not useful for diagnosis due to elevations in benign thyroid conditions. Recurrence or metastases are unlikely if thyroglobulin concentrations are less than 2 ng/mL with thyroid hormone suppression and less than 3 ng/mL without suppression. Anti-thyroglobulin antibodies, present in many thyroid carcinoma patients, interfere with the measurement of thyroglobulin. Therefore, the presence of antibodies should be determined prior to interpretation of thyroglobulin results.

In MTC, the production of calcitonin by the follicular C cells is used to confirm fine needle aspirate findings, to detect familial MTC through screening, to monitor treatment, and to detect disease recurrence. Calcitonin concentrations correlate with the extent of disease such as tumor volume. Higher levels are found in palpable disease while concentrations may be slightly elevated in normal or smaller tumors. Calcitonin concentrations also correlate with local and distant metastases. Sensitivity of calcitonin in detecting small tumors and C-cell hyperplasia is increased using stimulation with calcium and/or pentagastrin (table 2). In the calcium and pentagastrin combined test, 2 mg/kg of elemental calcium (20 mg/kg calcium gluconate) is given IV over 60 seconds followed by 0.5 μg/kg of pentagastrin over 5 to 10 seconds. Serum calcitonin concentrations are measured at 0, 1, 2, 3, 5, 7, 10 and 15 minutes. Concentrations rising to 200% over baseline are suggestive of MTC. A five fold elevation is often seen in MTC or C-cell hyperplasia when basal calcitonin concentrations are only slightly elevated. In sporadic or familial disease, calcitonin stimulation testing following treatment is the norm for monitoring recurrence and detecting residual disease.

Diagnosis of familial forms of MTC can be made before clinical or biochemical evidence with genetic testing as discussed in the section on MEN-2. Patients with apparent sporadic disease should be followed to determine the possibility of familial disease. Without bilateral disease, family history, or evidence of pheochromocytoma or hyperparathyroidism genetic testing is not indicated. A mutation in the index case necessitates screening of first degree family members with prophylactic thyroidectomies in gene carriers.

Other Tests. Fine needle aspiration with cytology is a primary diagnostic tool for distinguishing malignant and non-malignant disease, although this technique cannot distinguish all types of thyroid cancers. Immunohistochemical stains for calcitonin and chromagranin A are employed to diagnose MTC.

Tumor Imaging. Ultrasound and radionuclide scans are often part of the diagnostic work-up of thyroid nodules.

Breast, Ovarian, Prostate, and Testicular Malignancies

Breast Cancer

Epidemiology. Breast cancer leads all other cancers in new cancer cases in women in 1998 with 180,300 estimated cases and 43,900 estimated deaths. It is estimated that 1 in 8 women will be diagnosed with breast cancer during their lifetimes. In men, 1,600 new cancer cases and 400 deaths are estimated for 1998.

Risk and Hereditary Factors. The primary risk factor for breast cancer development is sex. In women other factors increasing risk include: age, previous history of breast cancer, family history of breast cancer, ionizing radiation exposure, increased exposure to estrogen and or progesterone, menarche earlier than 12 years, late menopause, age at first birth, history of specific benign breast disease (hyperplasia with atypia), diabetes mellitus, and alcoholic beverage use. In women, risk is decreased with lactation, early age at full term pregnancy, and physical activity. Approximately 5% of breast cancers have a genetic component. Mutations in *BRCA1*, *BRCA2*, *p53* and the androgen receptor genes (in men) have been associated with breast cancer. Li-Fraumeni syndrome, manifested by the development of breast cancer, sarcomas, and primary brain tumors, results from a germline mutation in the *p53* gene. In men, breast cancer risk is increased with Klinefelter's syndrome, gynecomastia, and a family history of male breast cancer.

Pathology. The histologic distribution of types of breast cancer is as follows: ductal adenocarcinoma (75%), lobular carcinoma (9%), comedocarcinoma (5%), medullary carcinoma (4%), colloid carcinoma (5%), and inflammatory carcinoma (1%). Metastases are to regional lymph nodes, the skin, bone, liver, lungs, and brain.

Clinical Features. Ninety percent of patients with breast cancer have detectable breast lumps. Spontaneous nipple discharge, skin changes, axillary lymphadenopathy, and symptoms of metastatic disease (bony pain, weight loss, and malaise) may also be present. The American Cancer Society recommendations include: monthly self exams in women over age 20, physical exams every 3 years for women ages 20-40 and annual exams over age 40; baseline mammograms between ages 35-39, repeat mammograms every 1-2 years between ages 40 49, and yearly mammograms after age 50.

Laboratory Tests. Currently, tumor markers for breast cancer are neither sensitive nor specific enough for screening or early detection of the disease. Carcinoembryonic antigen (CEA, reference range: <3 ng/mL), a cell surface glycoprotein also showing tumor marker utility for colorectal, GI, and lung cancer, has been used to monitor therapy of metastatic breast cancer and to detect bone or lung metastasis. However, CEA has recently been supplanted with more specific markers such as CA 15-3, CA 549, CA 27.29, and mucin-like carcinoma associated antigen (MCA).

The CA 15-3, CA 549, CA 27.29, and MCA antigens are high molecular weight mucins produced in mammary epithelium by the *MUC-1* gene. Production of monoclonal antibodies derived from sources such as milk-fat globules and human breast cancer cell lines have allowed the development of more specific tumor marker assays. Characteristics of these MUC-1 mucin monoclonal antibodies, such as epitope recognition, have been intensely studied. Despite some assay differences, the mucin based breast markers appear to have similar clinical performance.

The lack of ability of these markers to diagnose breast cancer is illustrated from a multicenter study of CA 549 in 237 women with breast cancer. When examined by stage, 5% of stage I, 14% of stage II, 32% of stage III, and 74% of stage IV patients were determined to have elevated CA 549 concentrations. Significant elevations were not noted for the lower stages. However, these markers are useful for monitoring therapy and disease progression in metastatic breast cancer patients. A change in CA

15-3 levels (>25%) correlates with disease progression in 80-90%, regression in 70-80%, and stable disease in 60-70% of patients. For detecting the recurrence of breast cancer, CA 27.29 has a sensitivity of 58%, a specificity of 98%, a positive predictive value of 83%, and a negative predictive value of 93%. In a recent study using the CA 27.29 marker, the lead time for predicting recurrence was 5.3 months. Despite a number of published studies showing potential clinical utility of serum tumor markers for breast cancer, an expert panel from the American Society of Clinical Oncology has declined to recommend the use of CEA, CA 15-3, or CA 27-29, citing a small body of evidence and lack of clinical benefit.

Tumor markers for breast cancer can also play a role in prognosis, identifying patients who may benefit from adjuvant treatment. These markers, reflecting specific features of the tumor, may be biochemical or molecular markers. Some of these markers include: hormone receptor status, DNA ploidy/S-phase fraction, HER-2/*neu* expression, *p53* tumor suppressor gene mutations, and cathepsin-D levels. The determination of hormone receptor (estrogen and progesterone) status, has been shown to be useful for prognosis and predicting response to hormonal therapy.

Other Tests. Following detection of a potentially malignant breast mass, fine needle aspiration cytology, excisional biopsy, cyst aspiration may be performed.

Tumor Imaging. Mammography is the most sensitive diagnostic technique for detecting breast cancer. Mammography detects 85% of breast cancers, 45% before they are palpable. Liver and bone scans are employed to detect metastatic disease.

Ovarian Cancer

Epidemiology. 25,400 new cases and 14,500 deaths from ovarian carcinoma are estimated for 1998. Ovarian cancer is the fifth leading cancer site accounting for 4% of cancers and 5% of cancer deaths. Peak incidence of the disease occurs in the eighth decade.

Risk and Hereditary Factors. Less than 5% of ovarian cancer is familial with a 50% increased risk with 2 or more first degree or second degree relatives with epithelial ovarian cancer. Inherited disease is manifested in an autosomal dominant fashion though three mechanisms: site-specific ovarian cancer (family ovarian cancer history), familial breast and ovarian cancer syndrome, and Lynch type II syndrome (family history of colorectal, endometrial, ovarian, pancreatic, and other cancers). Genes responsible for susceptibility for ovarian cancer include: *BRCA1*, *BRCA2*, and *HNPCC* (hereditary non-polyposis colon cancer). Late menopause and a personal history of breast or endometrial cancer also increases risk. The highest rates for ovarian cancer are in industrialized countries suggesting an environmental and/or dietary link. Use of oral contraceptives for over five years imparts a 50% reduced risk for ovarian cancer. Parity is also protective with a 70% decrease risk with 3 or more live births.

Pathology. Tumors are classified as epithelial (95%, majority are serous or mucinous adenocarcinoma), germ cell (2-3%), or sex cord stromal (2%). Metastases occur to the omentum, peritoneal surfaces, bowel mesentery, sigmoid colon, and retroperitoneal lymph nodes. Twenty to thirty percent of tumors in postmenopausal women and 7% in premenopausal women are malignant.

Clinical Features. There are no specific symptoms for ovarian cancer and early disease may be totally asymptomatic. The lack of specific symptoms contributes to the diagnosis of a majority of ovarian cancers at advanced stages. Non-specific symptoms include: irregular menses (premenopausal), urinary frequency, constipation, abnormal vaginal bleeding, abdominal discomfort, distention, and fatigue. Abdominal masses or ascites are suspicious for ovarian cancer. Early stage cancer may be discovered incidentally on routine pelvic exam.

Laboratory Tests. The tumor marker most useful for ovarian cancer is CA 125, a high-molecular mass glycoprotein expressed by epithelial ovarian tumors, and other pathological and normal tissues of Müllerian duct origin. In a healthy population the upper reference limit of CA 125 is 35 U/mL. CA 125 is not useful for screening asymptomatic populations as it is neither sensitive nor specific. CA 125 is elevated in other cancers such as endometrial, pancreatic, lung, breast, colorectal, and other GI tumors as well as in benign conditions such as cirrhosis, hepatitis, endometriosis, pericarditis, in early pregnancy, during menstruation, and in benign cysts. Approaches to improve the clinical utility of CA 125 for the early detection of ovarian cancer include using combinations of markers, increasing specificity by combining measurements with transvaginal ultrasonography, and monitoring changes in CA 125 concentrations over time.

CA 125 is elevated in most ovarian cancers; elevated values are seen in 50% of stage I disease and 90% of stage II to stage IV disease. Concentrations correlate with stage and tumor size. CA 125 is used to detect residual disease following initial therapy with a sensitivity of 50% and a specificity of 96%. CA 125 is 75% accurate in detecting recurrent metastases and correlates with disease progression or regression in 80-90%

of patients. In addition, CA 125 is indicative of prognosis following chemotherapy. A ten fold decrease after one cycle indicates a positive prognosis while no change after 3 cycles is indicative of a poor prognosis.

Additional tumor markers have been found to have utility in ovarian cancer. In contrast to CA 125 which is useful for epithelial tumors, human chorionic gonadotropin (β–hCG, reference range: <5 mIU/mL) and α–fetoprotein (AFP, reference range: <10 ng/mL) are most useful for germ cell tumors. In addition, CEA (reference range: <3 ng/mL) can be used to monitor response to therapy.

Other Tests. Other tests such as pelvic exams, Pap smears, and biopsies are employed for suspected cases of cancer.

Tumor Imaging. Ultrasound, both transabdominal and transvaginal, is a useful diagnostic tool. CT scans and MRI are also used, specifically to detect metastases.

Prostate Cancer

Epidemiology. 184,500 new cases of prostate cancer and 39,200 deaths are estimated for 1998. Of new cancer cases, prostate cancer is the leading site in men with 29% of cancers.

Risk and Hereditary Factors. There is an increased risk of prostate cancer with age, a greater risk in blacks compared to whites and, an increased risk with affected first degree relatives. In addition, diet is postulated to play a role in the etiology of prostate cancer. Ten percent of cancers are familial with one third of those estimated to have alterations in the recently discovered *HPC1* (hereditary prostate cancer 1) gene.

Pathology. The majority of prostate cancer tumors are adenocarcinomas. Metastases are primarily to the bone.

Clinical Features. With the exception of advanced disease, prostate cancer is usually asymptomatic. Abnormalities, physical induration or nodularity, on digital rectal exam (DRE) may represent prostate cancer. Symptoms of advanced disease, some as a result of metastases, include: urinary hesitancy or urgency, poor urine stream, dribbling, terminal hematuria, rapid onset urinary tract obstruction symptoms, bone pain, sudden paraplegia, and incontinence.

Laboratory Tests. PSA (prostate specific antigen), a serine protease produced by prostate epithelium, is the most effective tumor marker for prostate cancer although it is not highly sensitive or specific. Elevations in PSA (>4 ng/mL) may be due to benign prostate disease. PSA is used for early detection and for clinical management of prostate cancer.

PSA is combined with DRE for early detection to increase its clinical utility. The American Cancer Society recommends annual PSA testing and DRE for men over the age of 50 with at least a 10 year life expectancy and younger men at high risk. A number of approaches have been taken to increase the specificity of PSA, especially in the diagnostic gray zone of 4 to 10 ng/mL where there is overlap between prostate cancer and non-cancer. These approaches include age-specific reference ranges, PSA velocity, PSA density, neural network derived indexes, and measurement of the molecular forms of PSA.

The last approach, utilization of the molecular forms of PSA appears most promising. PSA is present in serum in a free form and complexed to protease inhibitors, primarily α_1-antichymotrypsin (ACT) and α_2-macroglobulin (A2M) although only free PSA and PSA-ACT are measured in total PSA assays. The majority of PSA in serum (80-90%) is in the complexed form although it has been observed that men with and without prostate cancer differ in the proportions of free PSA and PSA-ACT. Patients with prostate cancer have a lower percentage of free PSA (free PSA/total PSA) compared to those without cancer. A number of factors affect percent free PSA cutoffs, although it has been suggested that if percent free PSA is > 25% in men with a total PSA between 4 and 10 ng/mL the likelihood of prostate cancer is less than 10%, whereas if the percent free PSA is < 10% there is an 80% chance of cancer and a biopsy is recommended.

PSA correlates with clinical stages of prostate cancer, but is not reliable for use in individuals. PSA is most useful in monitoring response to therapy such as radical prostatectomy, radiation therapy, and antiandrogen therapy, and for detecting disease recurrence. Following definitive therapy, PSA concentrations are expected to reach undetectable concentrations if all prostatic tissue was surgically removed. Detectable post-prostatectomy PSA concentrations are indicative of local disease recurrence or distant metastases.

PAP (prostatic acid phosphatase) has been largely replaced by PSA as a tumor marker for prostate cancer. PAP is not sensitive for early cancer detection, however it is useful for staging of prostate cancer. This is due to elevations of PAP in 80-90% of patients with metastatic disease. PAP can be measured enzymatically or by immunoassay.

Other Tests. Transrectal ultrasound (TRUS) guided needle biopsies are used to diagnose prostate cancer.

Tumor Imaging. Tumors are imaged with TRUS and CT scans.

Testicular Cancer

Epidemiology. 7,600 new cases and 400 deaths from testicular cancer are estimated for 1998. Testicular cancer is the most common cancer in men ages 20 to 40.

Risk and Hereditary Factors. Males with cryptorchidism have 10 to 40 times increased risk of developing testicular cancer. Other risk factors include gonadal dysgenesis, Klinefelter's syndrome, and maternal use of diethystilbesterol (DES). The disease is 4.5 times more common in whites than in blacks.

Pathology. The majority of tumors (95%) in younger men arise from germ cells [seminomas (40-50%), embryonal and teratomas (50%), choriocarcinomas (<0.5%), and yolk sac tumors]. Cancers may be of one cell type or mixtures. Rhabdomyosarcoma, lymphoma, and melanoma comprise <5% of tumors. In men over age 60 lymphoma is most common. At diagnosis, 60% of tumors are localized, 24% are regional, and 14% are distant. Metastases are found in the lymph nodes, lungs, and liver.

Clinical Features. Commonly, testicular cancer is discovered as a painless enlargement by the patient. The diagnosis is subsequently made upon physical examination by the physician. Painful enlargements may be present in 30-50% of patients. Gynecomastia or infertility are primary symptoms in a small percentage of patients while the presence of back or flank pain may be indicative of metastases.

Laboratory Tests. Serum concentrations of human chorionic gonadotropin (hCG), a glycoprotein secreted by the synctiotrophoblastic cells of the normal placenta, and α-fetoprotein (AFP), a glycoprotein synthesized by the fetal yolk sac and liver during development, are valuable tumors for testicular cancer as either hCG or AFP or both are produced by 60-90% of non-seminomatous germ cell testicular tumors. Total β-hCG assays, measuring intact hCG and free β-subunits, may be preferable due to the production of free β-subunits in cancer.

Although β-hCG is present in 10% of seminomatous cases, a majority of embryonal germ cell tumors produce either β-hCG (>65%), AFP (>70%) or both. β-hCG is elevated in choriocarcinomas while AFP is elevated in yolk sac tumors. These markers are not useful for teratomas. Thus on suspicion of testicular cancer both markers are typically measured as diagnostic tools and for classifying tumor types. Elevations have been observed in <20% of patients with stage I, 50 to 80% with stage II, and 90 to 100% with stage III disease. Both markers have been found to correlate with tumor volume and disease prognosis and both markers are particularly useful for monitoring treatment response. Following orchiectomy, elevations in markers are indicative of residual, recurrent, or metastatic disease. Chemotherapy can also be monitored taking into account the half-lives of hCG (12-20 hours) or AFP (5 days).

Other tumor markers play a role in testicular cancers. Placental alkaline phosphatase, another oncodevelopmental marker, can be elevated in seminomas in addition to a number of other cancers. Sensitivity is increased when combined with the non-specific enzyme marker lactate dehydrogenase (LDH). LDH concentrations further correlate with tumor burden and therefore prognosis.

Tumor Imaging. Scrotal ultrasound can accompany physical diagnosis.

References

1. Landis SH, Murray T, Bolden S, Wingo PA. Cancer statistics 1998. CA Cancer J Clin 1997;48:6 29.
2. Chan DW, Sell S. Tumor markers. In: Burtis CA, Ashwood ER, eds. Tietz textbook of clinical chemistry, third ed. Philadelphia, PA: W.B. Saunders Company, 1999:722-749.
3. Wu L-T, Chahinian AP, Baylin SB, Thompson NW, Averbuch AD. Neoplasms of the neuroendocrine system. In: Holland JF, Bast Jr. RC, Morton DL, Frei III E, Kufe DW, Ralph R. Weichselbaum RR, eds. Cancer Medicine, 4th edition. Baltimore, MD: Williams & Wilkins, 1997:1571-1604.
4. Sizemore GW. Multiple endocrine neoplasia. In: Becker KL, ed. Principles and Practice of Endocrinology and Metabolism, second edition. Philadelphia: J. B. Lippincott Company, 1995:1555-64.
5. Wick MJ. Clinical and molecular aspects of multiple endocrine neoplasia. Clin Lab Med 1997;17:39-57.
6. Chandrasekharappa SC, Gurur SC, Manickam, et al. Positional cloning of the gene for multiple endocrine neoplasia-type 1. Science 1997;276:404-7.
7. Dawson DB, Jialal I. Multiple endocrine neoplasia. Diag Endocrinol Metab 1996;14:279-92.
8. Chanson P, Cadiot G, Murat A. Management of patients and subjects at risk for multiple endocrine neoplasia type 1: MEN 1. Horm Res 1997;47:211-20.

9. Bassett JHD, Forbes SA, Pannett AAJ, et al. Characterization of mutations in patients with multiple endocrine neoplasia type 1. Am J Hum Genet 1998;62:232-44.

10. Multiple endocrine neoplasia, type 2. Online mendelian inheritance in man (www3.ncbi.nlm.nih.gov/omim/).

11. Moley JF. The molecular genetics of multiple endocrine neoplasia type 2A and related syndromes. Ann Rev Med 1997;48:409-20.

12. Mazzaferri EL. Thyroid cancer. In: Becker KL, ed. Principles and Practice of Endocrinology and Metabolism, second edition. Philadelphia: J. B. Lippincott Company, 1995:354-66.

13. Baisen BL, Chan DW. Carcinoid syndrome. Diag Endocrinol Metab 1997;15:33-5.

14. O'Dorisio TM, Ellison EC, Johnson JA, Mazzaferri EL. Multiple endocrine neoplasia and gastrinoma. In: Mazzaferri EL, Samaan NA, eds. Endocrine tumors. Oxford: Blackwell Scientific Publications, 1993:484-96.

15. Henderson AR, Tietz NW, Rinker AD. Gastric, pancreatic and intestinal function. In: Burtis CA, Ashwood ER, eds. Tietz textbook of clinical chemistry, second ed. Philadelphia, PA: W.B. Saunders Company,1994:1576-1644.

16. Kaplan LM. Gastrointestinal endocrine tumors. In: Moore WT, Eastman RC, eds. Diagnostic endocrinology, second edition. St. Louis, MO: Mosby, 1996:439-50.

17. Tyler DS. Pancreatic endocrine tumors and multiple endocrine neoplasia. In: Berger DH, Feig BW, Fuhrman GM. The M.D. Anderson surgical oncology handbook. Boston: Little Brown and Company, 1995:239-58.

18. Yeo C. Neoplasms of the endocrine pancreas. In: Greenfield LJ, Mulholland MW, Oldham KT, Zelenock GZ, Lillemoe KD, eds. Surgery: scientific principals in practice, second ed. Philadelphia, PA: Lippincott-Raven Publishers, 1997.

19. Hammond PJ, Gibley SG, Wynick D, Bloom SR. Glucagonoma, VIPoma, somatostatinoma, other hormones, and nonfunctional tumors. In: Mazzaferri EL, Samaan NA, eds. Endocrine tumors. Oxford: Blackwell Scientific Publications, 1993:457-483.

20. Eastman RC. Hypoglycemia. In: Moore WT, Eastman RC, eds. Diagnostic endocrinology, second edition. St. Louis, MO: Mosby, 1996:229-42.

21. Sacks DB. Carbohydrates. In: Burtis CA, Ashwood ER, eds. Tietz textbook of clinical chemistry, second ed. Philadelphia, PA: W.B. Saunders Company, 1994:928-1001.
22. Field JB. Insulinoma. In: Mazzaferri EL, Samaan NA, eds. Endocrine tumors. Oxford: Blackwell Scientific Publications, 1993:497-530.
23. Carlson HE, Lowitz BB, Casciato DA. Endocrine neoplasms. In: Casciato DA, Lowitz BB, eds. Manual of clinical oncology, third edition. Boston: Little, Brown and Company, 1995:268-87.
24. Samaan NA, Schultz PN, Hickey RC. Adrenocortical carcinoma. In: Mazzaferri EL, Samaan NA, eds. Endocrine tumors. Oxford: Blackwell Scientific Publications, 1993:422-5.
25. D'Orisio MS, Qualman SJ. Neuroblastoma. In: Mazzaferri EL, Samaan NA, eds. Endocrine tumors. Oxford: Blackwell Scientific Publications, 1993:448-54.
26. Hurvitz CGH. Cancers in childhood. In: Casciato DA, Lowitz BB, eds. Manual of clinical oncology, third edition. Boston: Little, Brown and Company, 1995:318-23.
27. Keiser HR. Pheochromocytoma and other diseases of the sympathetic nervous system. In: Becker KL, ed. Principles and Practice of Endocrinology and Metabolism, second edition. Philadelphia: J. B. Lippincott Company, 1995:762-70.
28. Bravo EL, Gifford RW, Manger WM. Adrenal medullary tumors: pheochromocytoma. In: Mazzaferri EL, Samaan NA, eds. Endocrine tumors. Oxford: Blackwell Scientific Publications, 1993:426 47.
29. Mallette LE. Hyperparathyroidism. In: Mazzaferri EL, Samaan NA, eds. Endocrine tumors. Oxford: Blackwell Scientific Publications, 1993:625-70.
30. Silverberg SJ, Fitzpatrick LA, Bilezikian JP. Primary hyperparathyroidism. In: Becker KL, ed. Principles and Practice of Endocrinology and Metabolism, second edition. Philadelphia: J. B. Lippincott Company, 1995:512 20.
31. Blair EA, Barnes, Jr. G. Carcinoma of the thyroid and parathyroid glands. In: Berger DH, Feig BW, Fuhrman GM. The M.D. Anderson surgical oncology handbook. Boston: Little Brown and Company, 1995:275-292.

32. Samaan NA, Ordonez NG, Hickey RC. Medullary thyroid cancer. In: Mazzaferri EL, Samaan NA, eds. Endocrine tumors. Oxford: Blackwell Scientific Publications, 1993:334-47.

33. Moore WT, Eastman RC. Laboratory evaluation of diseases of the thyroid. In: Moore WT, Eastman RC, eds. Diagnostic endocrinology, second edition. St. Louis, MO: Mosby, 1996:177-209.

34. Cady B, Rolla AR. Neoplasms of the endocrine glands. In: Holland JF, Bast Jr. RC, Morton DL, Frei III E, Kufe DW, Ralph R. Weichselbaum RR, eds. Cancer Medicine, 4th edition. Baltimore, MD: Williams & Wilkins, 1997:1542-62.

35. Endres DB, Rude RK. Mineral and bone metabolism. In: Burtis CA, Ashwood ER, eds. Tietz textbook of clinical chemistry, second ed. Philadelphia, PA: W.B. Saunders Company, 1994:1887-1973.

36. Fisher B, Osborne CK, Margolese RG, Bloomer WD. Neoplsams of the breast. In: Holland JF, Bast Jr. RC, Morton DL, Frei III E, Kufe DW, Ralph R. Weichselbaum RR, eds. Cancer Medicine, 4th edition. Baltimore, MD: Williams & Wilkins, 1997:2349-2432.

37. Leach SD, Feig BW, Berger DH. Invasive breast cancer. In: Berger DH, Feig BW, Fuhrman GM. The M.D. Anderson surgical oncology handbook. Boston: Little Brown and Company, 1995:12-37.

38. Haskell CM, Casciato DA. Breast Cancer. In: Casciato DA, Lowitz BB, eds. Manual of clinical oncology, third edition. Boston: Little, Brown and Company, 1995:183-99.

39. Chan DW. Markers for breast cancer. AACC Endo 1995;13:71-3.

40. Summary report on the ISOBM TD-4 workshop: analysis of 56 monoclonal antibodies against the MUC1 mucin. Tumor Biol 1998;19(suppl 1):1-20.

41. Chan DW, Beveridge RA, Bhargava A, Wilcox PM, Kennedy MJ, Schwartz MK. Breast cancer marker CA549. A multicenter study. Am J Clin Path 1994;101:465-70.

42. Chan DW, Beveridge RA, Muss H, Fritsche HA, Hortobagyi G, Theriault R, Kiang D, Kennedy BJ, Evelegh M. Use of Truquant BR radioimmunoassay for early detection of breast cancer recurrence in patients with stage II and stage III disease. J Clin Oncol 1997;15:2322-8.

43. 1997 Update of recommendations for the use of tumor markers in breast and colorectal cancer. J Clin Oncol 1998;16:793-5.

44. Diamandis EP. Prognostic makers in breast cancer. Clin Lab News 1996;22:46-51.
45. Berek JS, Thomas GM, Ozols RF. Ovarian cancer. In: Holland JF, Bast Jr. RC, Morton DL, Frei III E, Kufe DW, Ralph R. Weichselbaum RR, eds. Cancer Medicine, 4th edition. Baltimore, MD: Williams & Wilkins, 1997:2289-2327.
46. Hallum AV, Coleman RL, Wolf J. Gynecologic oncology. In: Berger DH, Feig BW, Fuhrman GM. The M.D. Anderson surgical oncology handbook. Boston: Little Brown and Company, 1995:326-68.
47. Farias-Eisner RP, Walker DL, Berek JS. Gynecologic cancers. In: Casciato DA, Lowitz BB, eds. Manual of clinical oncology, third edition. Boston: Little, Brown and Company, 1995:200-27.
48. Boyce N. Successful strategies for tumor markers. Tumor markers of the future. Clin Lab News 1997;23:7.
49. Delworth MG, Dinney CP. Genitourinary cancer. In: Berger DH, Feig BW, Fuhrman GM. The M.D. Anderson surgical oncology handbook. Boston: Little Brown and Company, 1995:308-25.
50. Figlin RA, deKernion JB. Urinary tract cancers. In: Casciato DA, Lowitz BB, eds. Manual of clinical oncology, third edition. Boston: Little, Brown and Company, 1995:237-57.
51. Smith JR, Freije D, Carpten JD et al. Major susceptibility locus for prostate cancer on chromosome 1 suggested by a genome-wide search. Science 1996;274:1371-4.
52. Chan DW, Sokoll LJ. Prostate-specific antigen: update 1997. J Int Fed Clin Chem 1997;9:120-5.
53. Partin AW, Oesterling JE. The clinical usefulness of prostate specific antigen: update J Urol 1994;152:1358.
54. von Eschenbach A, Ho R, Murphy GP, Cunningham M, Lins N. American Cancer Society guidelines for the early detection of cancer. Cancer 1997;80:1805-7.
55. Partin AW, Carter HB. The use of prostate-specific antigen and free/total prostate-specific antigen in the diagnosis of localized prostate cancer. Urol Clin North Am 1996;23:531-40.
56. Einhorn LH, Lowitz BB. Testicular cancer. In: Casciato DA, Lowitz BB, eds. Manual of clinical oncology, third edition. Boston: Little, Brown and Company, 1995:228-36.

57. Nichols CR, Timmerman R, Foster RS, Roth BJ, Einhorn LH. Neoplasms of the testis. In: Holland JF, Bast Jr. RC, Morton DL, Frei III E, Kufe DW, Ralph R. Weichselbaum RR, eds. Cancer Medicine, 4th edition. Baltimore, MD: Williams & Wilkins, 1997:2177-2214.

Index

A

D

E

M

R

W

X

Z